STROKE

'*Stroke* is aimed at the victims and their carers. It starts with a concise summary of what a stroke is and how the patient is affected, then it progresses clearly through all possible stages – progression, regression and stasis – covering every aspect in a greater depth and breadth than might be expected. There simply isn't space here to do this book justice.'

Nursing Times

'If you hear of any book which claims to be a "Complete Guide", you may be forgiven for an initially sceptical reaction, but Laura Swaffield has produced such a book.'

Therapy Weekly

STROKE

THE COMPLETE GUIDE TO RECOVERY AND REHABILITATION

Laura Swaffield

Thorsons
An Imprint of HarperCollins*Publishers*

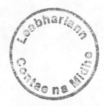

Thorsons
An Imprint of HarperCollins*Publishers*
77–85 Fulham Palace Road,
Hammersmith, London W6 8JB

First published by Thorsons 1990
This revised edition 1996
3 5 7 9 10 8 6 4 2

A catalogue record for this book
is available from the British Library

ISBN 0 7225 3241 5

Printed and bound in Great Britain by
Caledonian International Book Manufacturing Ltd, Glasgow

CONTENTS

CONSULTANTS ON SPECIALIST AREAS

Psychologist: Colin R. Brett BA MA DHP DipAdlCouns is a counsellor, psychotherapist, management consultant and counsellor trainer. He works in the UK, Eire, Germany and South Africa, and has played a leading role in the Adlerian Society of Great Britain.

Occupational therapist: Rose Lacey has worked as the specialist OT adviser to carers with the Sutton Carers Project run by the local authority in Sutton, England. She previously set up a stroke club, specialized in geriatrics and developed the concept of individualized 'care packages'.

Speech therapist: Deborah Rossiter is former professional speech therapy adviser to the British charity ADA (Action for Dysphasic Adults), and Ruth Coles MSc MRCSLT is ADA's current speech therapy adviser and director. Both have long experience with stroke patients and carers, mainly in the UK's National Health Service.

Physiotherapist: Pamela Grasty BA MCSP DipTP is former superintendent physiotherapist at Brighton General Hospital, England and Ann Holland MCSP Grad Dip Phys is clinical physiotherapist at the Neurorehabilitation Unit, National Hospital for Neurology and Neurosurgery.

FOREWORD

As this book reveals, stroke is a common, killing and disabling disease. About 70,000 deaths each year are due to stroke which places it third in the mortality statistical tables after heart disease and cancer. It leads the list of seriously disabling conditions. Its very suddenness transforms personal and family life at a stroke.

Yet stroke is a neglected disease. It does not get to the public heart as do some much less common, perhaps more exotically named diseases. Indeed the medical profession at large finds it difficult to maintain enthusiasm for stroke. This may be due to the lack, as yet, of a definitive drug treatment to arrest or reverse the immediate effects of the disease; a perception that it affects only older people and that nothing very effective can be done to help nature in the recovery period.

But doctors do not have the monopoly in stroke treatment. Those who appreciate the need for a team effort involving nurses, therapists – physio, occupational and speech – produce the best results and certainly can claim the most contented patients. It seems common sense that such teams can best operate in specialized stroke units.

No matter how excellent a hospital-based stroke service may be, however, there is invariably a great gap to be bridged when the stroke person returns home. Community-based services are patchy and invariably inadequate. This book will help to fill that gap. Intended to give sympathetic advice and information to carers and others as well as those stricken by stroke it is extremely comprehensive. All aspects of prevention, treatment, rehabilitation and long-term recovery care are covered. Advice to stroke sufferers exhorts them not to give up; recovery can continue for longer periods than previously accepted wisdom would have us believe and an optimistic view of the future is rightly encouraged. To friends and colleagues goes the needed reminder that intelligence is not lost in stroke; patients should not therefore be treated as though it had.

The carer's role should not involve doing too much for the stroke person; he or she must be encouraged to work for their own recovery. Carers must look after their own physical and mental health so that their vital roles are not prejudiced by ill health. The carer is encouraged by Laura Swaffield to cooperate with professionals and this is sound advice.

This book will certainly serve as a valuable reference work and make fascinating reading for concerned carers.

Sir David Atkinson KBE, FRCPE, FFCM, FFOM
Former Director General, The Chest, Heart and Stroke Association

INTRODUCTION

This book is for anyone whose life has suddenly been turned upside down by a stroke. Perhaps the stroke has happened to you; perhaps it has happened to someone you know. Either way, you deserve some help.

The good news is that enormous progress has been made in stroke rehabilitation. Many stroke survivors today are making recoveries which would have been thought impossible even a few years ago.

No two strokes are the same. Some are minor, and wear off almost completely. Some are severe, with lasting effects. These effects also vary: different physical signs, different emotional reactions.

The important thing is to find out as much as you can about *this* stroke, and the impact it is likely to have on *your* life. Then you can start to get a grip on your situation. It may not look too good at first, but understanding your own individual problems is the first step towards solving them. This book aims to help you do exactly that.

Once you know where you are, and where you want to get to, rehabilitation can become an interesting project rather than something you just 'cope with' in a passive way.

The book is arranged in clear, separate sections. You'll want to dip into the sections which mean most to you, and you'll need to look ahead and be prepared for changes. It's also a good idea to look back sometimes: to make sure you remember the important bits, to see if you missed something the first time round that has suddenly become relevant now.

This is a very basic book. It's a good start. You can be certain you'll need more detailed information about all kinds of things that specially concern you. And you are certain to find it: from the professionals you meet, and from the organizations listed at the back. Never be afraid to ask!

Getting back in control can be hard work, both for the stroke patient and for those who care for him or her. Don't underestimate the problems – but don't underestimate your powers to come up with solutions which suit you as an individual.

1

BASIC FACTS

What is a stroke?

Like everything else in the body, the brain depends on a constant supply of blood to keep it going. If the blood supply is cut off for four minutes or more, brain cells start to die. This is what happens with a stroke.

A stroke happens very suddenly – at a stroke. Only a minority – about 5 per cent – take up to a week to complete their effects. Just what those effects are depends on how many brain cells die, and exactly where they are in the brain.

About 30 per cent of stroke victims die within about three weeks, most of them on the first day. The rest will all recover to some extent, either quickly or slowly. Many patients recover completely. *(Note:* it is also possible for a long series of 'mini-strokes' to destroy brain function progressively, leading to dementia. This tragedy is outside the scope of this book.)

Some 'strokes' wear off completely, within minutes or hours. These episodes are called 'transient ischaemic attacks' (TIAs) and are a very serious warning that a full stroke will happen unless action is taken to prevent it. There is a separate explanation of TIAs on page 17.

Strokes only rarely cause pain. About 20 per cent of patients have a stroke in their sleep, and know nothing about it until they wake up. The brain itself is completely incapable of feeling pain.

Most patients are fully conscious while they have their strokes. About a third lose consciousness. These are often, but not always, the most serious cases. Up to half of all patients become mildly confused or drowsy, although it is so natural to feel confused in the circumstances that it is hard to tell when there is clinical confusion. The carer probably feels pretty confused as well. Both patient and carer will be very frightened.

There is no immediate danger. The patient does not have to be rushed off to hospital in an ambulance although patients who are unconscious are more likely to be sent to hospital right away. He or she may not need to go to hospital at all. This does not mean he or she is not expected to recover. Medical treatment may not be needed; *emergency* medical treatment is needed only very rarely.

Medical tests, however, will be made to confirm that a stroke really has happened, and to find out why it happened, how bad it is and whether treatment is required to prevent a further stroke. Only about 10 per cent of patients have another stroke within a year, once they have got through the first three weeks.

The way to make the best possible recovery is to work on rehabilitation. That is the main focus of this book, and it can achieve wonders. Some patients recover all by themselves; others have to work very hard – and so do those who care for them. It is worth it. The sooner the rehabilitation starts, the greater the chance of a full recovery.

Nobody can tell how serious any stroke is until tests are made, and a few days have passed. In the first few days, part of the brain begins to recover by itself, and the patient may improve rapidly. Then progress slows down. After a few months, professionals can estimate how much more progress the patient will be likely to make, given the progress so far. It is only an estimate. It is not at all unusual for stroke patients and their carers to take the pessimists by surprise.

The message: rehabilitation may be hard work, and it may be frustrating and tiring. But it is worth doing.

(*Note:* the word 'patient' is used in this book because it is the simplest word. But stroke survivors do not need to be babied: the more independent they get, and the sooner they do it, the better. Remember this!)

What causes a stroke?

A stroke happens when the blood supply to the brain is cut off. But how does the blood supply get cut off?

THROMBOSIS

This is the commonest cause of strokes – over half of them. The blood is thick and sluggish, and a clot (thrombus) forms. This blocks up the artery, and the blood flow stops. If there is a damaged spot on the artery wall, as there often is, the clot is likely to form at that spot. The damage to the artery wall is caused by a condition called atherosclerosis.

EMBOLUS

This is the next commonest cause, and it is very like thrombosis.

An embolus is just a thrombus (clot) which has formed somewhere else in the body – not in the artery to the brain where it finally arrives (and cuts off the blood supply). It may, for instance, form in the heart after a heart attack, and travel up to the brain.

Atherosclerosis

This word is a mixture of two words which mean separate things: arteriosclerosis and atheroma. Arteriosclerosis is 'hardening of the arteries' – artery walls which are coated with blood fat, cholesterol and/or calcium. This makes them stiff and narrow. Blood pulses strongly to force its way through, leading to high blood pressure and damage to the artery walls.

The mixture of deposits on the artery walls is called atheroma. Sometimes a piece breaks off and travels along the artery to become an embolus somewhere else (such as the brain). Blood which makes atheroma deposits is likely to be thick and fatty – the kind that can turn into a thrombus (clot). The thrombus is likely to form, or get stuck, at a damaged spot on the artery wall, because it will be roughened and will tend to catch on things.

Obviously, if the cause of the stroke is thrombus or embolus, you are pretty sure of finding atherosclerosis in the arteries. All three may happen together. You are also likely to find high blood pressure. Bringing down high blood pressure is one of the most important things people can do to prevent strokes.

CEREBRAL HAEMORRHAGE

This means brain bleeding. It causes about 15 per cent of strokes. There is a sudden burst in an artery wall under pressure – rather like a bursting tyre. Blood spurts out into the brain, causing a damaging rise in pressure, while the blood in the artery forms a clot which blocks off the supply of fresh blood.

The burst may be caused by high blood pressure. Or it may take place at a part of the artery wall which has always been weak (this is called an aneurysm). Urgent surgery may be needed to stop the leakage and repair the aneurysm.

These strokes, then, are the ones which justify an urgent trip to hospital. It is easy to tell them apart from the more usual, painless strokes caused by thrombosis and embolus (clots). Cerebral haemorrhages nearly always cause severe head pain – quite unlike any headaches the patient has had before. Severe head pain is always worth getting to hospital. If it is not a haemorrhage, it could be something equally serious, like meningitis.

What are the effects of a stroke?

No two strokes are alike. What happens will depend on (i) how much permanent damage has been done to the brain and (ii) where the damage happened.

The brain has two sides – right and left. Confusingly enough, the right side of the brain controls the left side of the body, and vice versa. A stroke in the left side of the brain will show up on the right side of the body; a stroke in the right side of the brain will show up on the left side of the body.

One important point: the left side of the brain usually controls people's speech. If the stroke is in the left side of the brain, the patient will not only have damage to the right side of his body, but may lose some (or all) of his ability to understand words. This is much more frightening than the effects on the body.

A great deal of the brain controls movement. So, wherever the stroke has taken place in the brain, 90 per cent of patients will have some kind of trouble with movement. The

most common effect is called hemiplegia – half-paralysis.
One side of the body is more or less paralysed. At first, it is
weak and floppy (flaccid). If the effect is mild, it is called
hemiparesis.

Then there are all kinds of other, often very upsetting,
effects on the brain's functions. It varies a lot from patient
to patient, depending on where their brains have been damaged. There may be strange changes in vision, touch, judgement – even in the way the patient thinks.

The final, major effect should be taken very seriously
indeed – emotional damage. The patient is in a state of
shock. He is frightened, and possibly helpless. He may not
be able to understand a word anybody is saying. He may
well realize he has had a stroke – an idea which frightens
most people. He may have no idea what has happened to
him – equally frightening. He does not know if he is going
to die.

As he becomes more conscious of his surroundings, he
becomes aware of all kinds of even more frightening things.
He may not be able to see straight, or feel, or work out
where he is. Worst of all, he may not be able to think
straight. If he cannot understand words, he is even more
bewildered and frightened. He has probably never heard of
these little-known effects of stroke. He thinks he is going
mad. He is not; his intelligence is just the same, too. But he
is trapped in an unfamiliar body and brain.

The person nearest to the patient is in almost as bad a
state. She knows more or less what has happened – but
nobody can yet tell her what this will do to the patient.
Nobody knows that. The patient may die.

The carer suffers all the fears the patient feels, as the
effects of the stroke are revealed. Unless somebody takes
the trouble to explain things to her, she will know as little

as the patient does about what is going on. She may be devastated to find that the patient cannot speak to her, or even understand her. And all the more subtle effects on vision, thinking and so on make the patient behave strangely.

The carer, at least, does not directly suffer the effects of the stroke, as the patient does. She suffers something else – an overwhelming sense of panic and responsibility. If you are in such a situation, turn to the end of this section to find out what to do.

The effects in detail

About half of all strokes lead to permanent problems of some kind. They may be mild or severe.

- Up to 80 per cent of patients suffer hemiplegia (weakness on one side of the body).
- About half of all patients have slurred speech, although this often wears off quickly.
- About half of all patients have dysarthria (weak, drooping facial muscles), although this also often wears off quickly.
- A third of patients have dysphasia (loss of the ability to understand words). This may be mild or severe.
- About a third of patients have dysphagia (inability to swallow). This can wear off quickly, but when it persists it can be quite a problem.
- About a quarter of patients have disturbances to their sense of touch. This can cause blunted senses, clumsy movements, or inability to know where a limb is without looking at it. Complete loss of sensation is rare.
- Nearly all patients feel depressed after a stroke. This is hardly surprising. But a quarter of patients have severe, clinical depression, which can be helped by medication.

- About 7 per cent of patients have disturbances to their vision, such as partial or complete loss of sight in one eye. They simply cannot see half of what is in front of them – the half which matches the affected side of their body. Sometimes this effect goes even further. They are not aware that side of things exists at all. They ignore everything on that side – even their own body!
- About 2 per cent suffer a very unpleasant shooting or throbbing pain called 'thalamic' or 'central' pain. It may affect half the body, or only a small part. Drugs can help.

Other common problems include:

- anosognosia – the patient is unable to recognize one side of her body as her own. She may ignore it completely, or even think somebody else is in bed with her.
- ataxia – the patient is unable to co-ordinate her movements. This may affect her speech muscles, too, causing incomprehensible speech.
- apraxia – the patient, bafflingly, cannot do things if she wants to do them. She is physically capable of making the required movement, but she can only do it by chance. If she thinks about it, she cannot do it. This can happen with speech as well as movement.
- spatial distortion – the patient has lost her appreciation of space and dimensions. She cannot find her way round, she cannot judge distances, and so on.
- poor memory and concentration – the patient forgets things very quickly. She may not be able to get to the end of a sentence without forgetting what the beginning of it was. It is not always as serious as this, but the patient may find it very hard to concentrate on even the simplest things.

- impaired judgement – the patient shows a sort of lack of common sense. Her taste in clothes may become poor, she may do stupid things she would never have done before. But she is as intelligent as ever in every other respect.
- slowness – the patient becomes a very slow thinker, and often a rigid and stubborn one, too.

A maddening world

A stroke is a major crisis for anyone. For some patients, it is also a sudden plunge into a nightmarish, Alice in Wonderland world where nothing normal can be relied on.

Everyone knows that strokes usually leave patients with weakness or paralysis on one side. Most people know there are speech problems sometimes, although they probably don't know much about them. Most people *don't* know about the visual and sensory problems which can happen. The results can be bizarre and very hard to understand. For instance, let's take an ordinary hair brush – a common, harmless object which can be identified and used by anyone from a jet-setting executive to an Amazonian Indian. But not, possibly, by a stroke patient ...

- Mr A sees it, knows what it's for, but can't for the life of him think what it is called. He cries or shouts with frustration.
- Mrs B calls it a hair-vruth, or something similar, because she can't control her speech muscles. She sounds slurry and drunken, and probably feels embarrassed.
- Miss C calls it a gerbil, a floo-ja, or all kinds of other things, and is angry or upset at your inability to understand. She has no idea she is using the wrong word, or a non-word.

- Mr D wants to use the brush, but comes out with a 'telegram' which doesn't get through, like: 'She brought – it's mine ...'
- Mr E hasn't the slightest idea what it is, or what it's for.
- Mrs F knows what it's for, and has the strength to use it, but somehow when she deliberately sets out to pick it up, she can't. The more she tries, the more upset she gets.
- Miss G grasps it, but insists on trying to use it upside-down, or with the bristles facing outwards. She has to be gently corrected – every single time.
- Ms H simply does not know it is there. It is on her weak side, where she can't see anything at all.
- Mr I can see it held in his weak hand, and wonders indignantly who has got hold of his hair brush. He cannot understand that the hand holding the brush is his.

We could probably get to the end of the alphabet with equally strange examples. To the carer, the patient seems to be stupid, lazy, awkward or simply mad. And it is almost impossible to imagine what it's like for the patient. A frequent comment is: 'I thought I was going mad'.

You both need to know that these extraordinary events are, in fact, quite normal and a result of damage to the brain. You need to find out just what the problems are for this particular patient, so you are not battling against a total unknown. The doctor and the speech therapist are the most helpful professionals to ask.

Tests

Nearly all stroke patients will have some kind of medical testing. Usually, it is obvious that a stroke has taken place, but occasionally tests may be needed to make sure it was not an epileptic fit, or an early sign of a brain tumour (a third of all brain tumours can be successfully relieved by surgery), or other diseases like migraine, Parkinson's disease or multiple sclerosis.

If doctors agree that a stroke has taken place, it may still be necessary to carry out tests to make sure the cause is not cerebral haemorrhage. In most cases, a cerebral haemorrhage is obvious. But in other cases (especially in young patients) doctors may see signs that make them want to be sure. Whatever the cause of the stroke, doctors may also 'scan' the brain to see where the stroke has taken place, how big the area of damage is and/or how the blood flow within the brain has been affected. The most likely test is a CAT scan (computerized axial tomography). The patient's head is surrounded by a large machine which takes pictures of the damage. It is completely painless.

The patient may be wired up to an electrocardiograph machine (ECG) to take readings from the heart and detect any underlying heart disease. Again, this is completely painless. For all patients, the most important test is the simplest – to detect high blood pressure. This is a major cause of stroke. If it is not corrected, there may well be another stroke.

Sometimes, the arteries themselves will be investigated. There are various techniques, which may involve passing a tiny tube (catheter) into the artery and/or injecting a sort of dye which will show up the shape of the artery in an X-ray.

Most common of all are blood tests. A high blood

glucose level may reveal underlying diabetes, and high blood fats indicate thickened red blood and/or atherosclerosis. There may be an excess of red blood cells, changing the consistency of the blood. These conditions will have to be treated, to prevent any chance of further strokes.

Various other tests may be made, some very simple and some quite sophisticated. Practice varies from place to place and, of course, from stroke to stroke.

Medical treatment for stroke

Often, there is no medical treatment for stroke. The stroke has done its damage once and for all, and the job to do now is rehabilitation. Do not feel cheated if you are not offered medical treatment: it may not be needed.

Cerebral haemorrhage may need surgery, to repair the damage to the artery wall and make sure further damage is prevented.

In the more common types of stroke, those caused by blood clots (thrombus or embolus), treatment may include surgery to remove the remains of the clot. In all cases, there will be treatment to make the blood less likely to clot in future. Various drugs are used, with the general name of 'anti-coagulants' (anti-clotting agents), and the patient may have to take them for the rest of his life. Aspirin is very effective. Advice on diet may also be needed – a diet high in fats is not much help for thickened, fatty blood or for atheroma deposits on the artery walls.

If the patient has high blood pressure (and this is quite likely), drugs may be prescribed to bring it down. Again, the patient may have to take these for the rest of his life. Advice on diet and exercise will also be needed.

If the patient is made more or less immobile by the

stroke, a whole new group of dangers arise, caused by the immobility itself rather than by the stroke. These dangers include chest infections and pressure sores (see Section 3). There is also, rather more rarely, a danger that blood clots will form in the legs and cause another embolus which could travel to the lungs. Special stockings may be prescribed, or possibly drugs. All these dangers will fade away as the patient becomes more mobile.

Treatment for stroke is developing all the time, so you may find other techniques being used. None of them, however, can 'cure' the damage already done. They may, however, help to preserve surrounding cells which are still alive, and to prevent further strokes from happening. Several drugs are now on trial, including 'clot-busters' to clear any remaining tiny blood clots, drugs to increase the blood flow around the damaged part of the brain, drugs to limit the extent of the damage and drugs to stimulate brain function. Watch this space!

Complementary therapies

Complementary therapies, sometimes called alternative therapies, are increasingly popular. Some doctors disapprove of them totally, because the way they work cannot be explained in conventional medical terms. But they do work, and there is no reason why they should not work for stroke patients – and, indeed, for carers under stress.

You must bear several things in mind. Complementary therapies should be used as well as, not instead of, conventional medical treatment. You may not like drugs much, but they can be life-savers. You also need to check with the doctor that the stroke is fully completed, and is not one of the minority of strokes which continues to do damage for some days.

Above all, be very sure that the complementary therapist you choose is not a quack. Distrust a therapist who makes wild claims about instant results, or tries to turn you against medical treatment. Make absolutely sure he is not only well qualified in his field, but very experienced too. Strokes are not to be fooled about with.

You may find a good therapist who has no recognized qualification (especially if he or she is a spiritual healer rather than someone who gives physical treatment). But you are much, much better off with a therapist who does hold a recognized qualification. Take advice from the Institute for Complementary Medicine or the American Holistic Medical Association.

All complementary therapies have one thing in common: they work to treat the individual patient, not the disease. They work to increase, and balance, the patient's own power to heal himself. But treatment has a better chance if it starts as soon as it is medically safe. Although some small results may well be felt straightaway, good results will probably take a long time, and cost quite a lot of money. Almost any kind of complementary therapy may have good effects, but some of the more likely ones are as follows.

AROMATHERAPY

Massage with scented oils, carefully chosen by a properly qualified practitioner, is not just pleasant. It is a powerful treatment that can reduce pain, boost the body's recovery powers, soothe the emotions, relax and invigorate.

ACUPUNCTURE

This works by gauging the patient's 'energy flow' around the body. By placing needles at the right point, the acupuncturist corrects blocks and imbalances, and releases the patient's own power to heal herself. Acupuncture can also relieve pain.

REFLEXOLOGY
By massaging the foot, the reflexologist can treat both the brain itself and the body parts which have been affected by the stroke, helping to restore both feeling and function. Each part of the body is represented by a point on the foot.

HOMOEOPATHY
This treatment, used by the British Royal Family, employs natural substances in tiny, tiny doses to support the patient's inbuilt coping powers. The homoeopath will want to know all about the patient's temperament as well as his medical symptoms.

MEDICAL HERBALISM
Plant extracts, in herb teas, foods and tinctures taken by the spoonful, can help restore damaged circulation, thin down sluggish blood, heal and relax damaged blood vessels, support the nervous system and have a general calming effect.

COUNSELLING
Talking out problems will, obviously, be more of a frustration than a help to a patient who can't handle words any more. But it will be very valuable to other patients – and to carers – to be able to talk out fears, frustrations and the kind of anger and resentment which is only too natural, but hard to express to your nearest and dearest. When just chatting to someone is not enough help, call in an expert like a counsellor.

Recovery

If the patient does not die from the stroke, she will recover. Many patients recover completely. Others have to work hard to regain their lost functions, and some will be left with a lasting handicap of some kind. When a stroke first happens, it is impossible to predict just how fast – and how far – any individual patient will recover. It's possible there may be a second stroke, but as the days go by this becomes less and less likely.

The first few weeks show the fastest improvement. Brain cells which have died, of course, never recover. But brain cells just outside the main damage area may be only temporarily damaged, and will heal. Brain cells further outside the main damage area may be put out of action at first by local leakage and swelling. As these fade away, they come back to complete function. So there may be quite a lot of 'spontaneous recovery', which needs no help from outside.

After that, things slow down. To a limited extent, other brain cells might be able to take over some of the work done by the permanently damaged ones. Good therapy will work to make the best use of undamaged brain cells to do the job a different way. The patient will gradually learn confidence, which makes a lot of difference to what she can do. And finally, she will learn new ways to get round the disabilities which will never go away. All these things are part of the recovery process, and it can be hard to tell which is which. Only one thing is for sure: therapy and rehabilitation *work*. The effort put into them will pay off.

A few things can be predicted:

• Legs tend to recover better than arms, because they only have to make rather large, uncomplicated movements.

Fine arm and hand movements are less easy to bring back.

- Long-held skills, memories and words come back before those which have been more recently acquired.
- Strong motivation helps recovery. Building up the patient's optimism and self-esteem is important.
- The earlier treatment and therapy start, the better will be the eventual recovery. Physiotherapy may even start when the patient is still unconscious!

Transient ischaemic attacks (TIAs)

TIAs are very common, They are mini-strokes, caused by tiny blood clots which cause minimal damage. The effects wear off completely, usually in minutes rather than hours. Sometimes, they can take a day to wear off completely.

In themselves, TIAs are nothing to worry about. It's thought that many people have TIAs which are so small they cause no symptoms at all, and one person may have many such TIAs with no noticeable effects.

But they are a very serious warning that a more severe stroke might happen. If the blood can make a tiny clot, it can also make a bigger clot. Early treatment could well prevent a true stroke from happening.

First, get to your doctor. He will test your blood pressure. He will almost certainly prescribe aspirin (in a low dose, up to 300mg). Take it faithfully. It really does reduce your risk of a stroke.

Next, go through the next section on *Stroke prevention*. Take it very seriously!

Never, never neglect an incident which seems to be like a stroke, no matter how quickly and completely it goes away. Eyes are particularly sensitive to lack of oxygen in the brain, so a common symptom may be blurred vision, or even a temporary loss of vision lasting a minute or so.

Other symptoms mirror those of a true stroke: weakness or paralysis on one side of the body (sometimes the arm is affected but not the leg), dizziness, confusion, muddled speech, inability to think straight, loss of sensation or a sudden fall, hearing loss, a sudden inability to swallow, memory loss, nausea.

It is tempting to forget all about such bizarre little episodes – after all, they are all over in a few minutes. Don't ignore them. You are lucky to have had a warning. Act on it.

Stroke prevention

Strokes are very common – about 110,000 a year in the UK, 415,000 a year in the USA. That means, very roughly, that every five minutes somebody, somewhere, is having a stroke. Yet it is estimated that about half of all strokes could be prevented, using current knowledge.

Whether you have had a TIA, a first stroke or no symptoms at all, it is well worthwhile knowing how strokes can be prevented. As a bonus, the rules for preventing strokes are very much the same as those for preventing heart disease. (Heart disease can, of course, cause a stroke in itself if a heart attack causes a blood clot which travels on to block a brain artery.)

The main preventable causes of stroke are as follows

HIGH BLOOD PRESSURE
This is a major factor, putting strain on the artery walls. Often, people suffer from high blood pressure and feel no symptoms at all. So it is worth getting a regular check from

your family doctor (especially if you are over 65), and taking his advice seriously.

Drugs may be needed to control high blood pressure, and they will have to be taken for life. If your doctor says your blood pressure has now come back to normal, this does *not* mean you should stop the treatment. Do keep taking the tablets! Many people stop taking them because they have unpleasant side-effects. Don't make this potentially disastrous mistake. Go back to the doctor and try another drug. There is sure to be one that suits you.

Sometimes, high blood pressure can be controlled by some of the actions listed below, most of which are also good for the heart:

EXERCISE

Don't lose the habit of exercise, even if you are getting older. Even a regular brisk walk can make all the difference to your blood pressure (and your heart, too). Don't take up strenuous exercise all of a sudden if you have lost the habit, but work back gradually into a higher level of activity.

SMOKING

It is never too late to give up smoking, or at the very least to cut it down. It may not be easy, but you are guaranteed a healthier heart and lungs, and better blood pressure. Smoking definitely increases the risk of a stroke.

SALT

Some people are particularly susceptible to the effects of too much salt on their blood pressure. You don't know whether you are one of these people or not, so why take the risk? Almost anyone can cut down salt intake quite painlessly. Don't cook with salt, or sprinkle it automatically on food – taste, and then add the minimum. Try using a salt substitute – many people can't tell the difference. Cut down on processed foods, many of which contain a lot of salt even if they don't taste salty.

HEAVY DRINKING

There are lots of reasons why excessive alcohol ruins lives. The fact that it has a strong connection to stroke is just one more. It isn't always easy to admit that you drink too much, but it isn't easy having a stroke, either.

OVERWEIGHT

This isn't good for blood pressure or the heart. Cut down on fats (see below) and sugar. Cut down on processed foods, which are likely to contain a lot of both. Eat lots of high fibre foods, fruit and vegetables. Substitute white meat and fish for red meat. Eat just a little less. Exercise just a little more. And find pleasures other than eating when you feel like a treat! Small changes, added together, can make a lot of difference.

FATS IN THE DIET

These should be your special target. Not only are they a major cause of overweight, they may also build up in the blood and lead to atherosclerosis and/or thickened, sticky blood. Cut down on frying and grill or boil instead. Cut fat off meat and remove skin from poultry. Spread a little less on your bread, and switch to a low-fat spread. Roast meat on a rack to drain off the fat, and blot cooked foods with kitchen paper. Avoid 'browning' foods in fat, and cook with the absolute minimum of oil or fat to prevent food from sticking.

Not every stroke can be prevented. But many can. The

simple precautions listed above do not demand a great deal of effort, and other books can give you plenty of extra advice in carrying them out. The result will most certainly be better health and well-being, a healthier heart – and a maximum chance of avoiding stroke. Prevention is far, far better than cure.

DIABETES

If you are diabetic you are at an increased risk of stroke. All the actions outlined above will help, but the main thing is to keep your diabetes well controlled. Stick to the insulin, drugs or other routines prescribed. If they don't suit you, get medical advice and find a regime that does suit you.

Adding up the risks

Be aware that all these risk factors add up in quite a dramatic way. For instance, someone with high blood pressure has a four fold risk of stroke. A smoker has double the risk. But someone who has high blood pressure *and* smokes has 12 times the risk!

2

FIRST SHOCK

You want to help. This section has plenty of practical ideas for the first few hours or days after a stroke. First, look over the first chapter so you have a good idea of what has happened in medical terms and what is likely to happen next. Next, think about yourself ...

How do you feel?

A stroke is devastating. The suddenness with which it happens gives it emotional power equivalent to a major accident. Today it is taken for granted that counselling should be provided for survivors of major accidents, and for those involved in their rescue. Such counselling commonly goes on for months and years. Flashbacks, nightmares, depression, lack of confidence, tears or bursts of anger are, in the same way, understood to be likely to go on for months or years.

It's much the same with stroke. You'll probably need the same kind of support – but you're much less likely to get it offered on a plate.

Your first reaction will be just plain shock – numbness, blankness, a sense of unreality. This is a sort of natural pain-killing device, and it has its uses. Both patient and carer will feel it, because both have suffered a major loss. Loss of power over their lives. Loss of the patient's former self. Loss of plans for the future, which will have to change. Loss of freedom.

The carer will probably be pretty busy at this time, especially if the patient if being cared for at home. This also helps to keep feelings suppressed. The patient, of course, has much more time on his hands. Apart from the same sense of shock, he may have had damage to the brain which puts him in a doubly unreal world – vision or perception disturbance, confusion, exhaustion, depression.

The feeling of shock won't prevent emotional outbursts, in either of you. The first few days of a stroke are an unusually frightening time because you cannot be sure just what your situation is. There is no medical way to predict how well the patient is going to recover or, indeed, whether he'll survive the first weeks at all. No wonder you don't feel much, behind the tears and the upsets. You don't even know exactly what you've got to have feelings about.

GET EMOTIONAL SUPPORT

- **Seek comfort.** Sudden bad news breaks down barriers. It gives a sort of permission for touching and hugging between people who never normally do these things. Take advantage. The patient will be in need of touch to assure him he is still loved despite his new helplessness. If the patient has lost the power of speech or of understanding, his need is ten times more.
- **If you want to cry, cry.** Suppressed emotions make people ill. Don't waste energy cultivating a stiff upper lip. You'll need all the energy you can get.

- **Talk.** You need a sympathetic person who is prepared to *listen*, or as many such people as you can lay your hands on. There are no rules about where to find suitable people: it could be a friend or relative, a nurse, a priest or counsellor, a help-line – or the man in the corner shop! What you are looking for is someone who doesn't interrupt, doesn't tell you what they think, and doesn't give you well-meaning advice. What will do you good is getting your fears and feelings aired – your output, not somebody else's input. A pet animal can make a perfectly adequate listener. It will have more patience than a human and, at this stage, its opinions will have just as much value!

Get your feet on the ground

This emotional work is the most valuable work you can do, but you'll probably have an urge to keep busy which you'll need to exploit as well. Start reading some of the later sections in this book to get an idea of the kind of things you may need to organize.

Find out all you can, as soon as anything is known. Almost as soon as the stroke is over, professionals will start to note exactly what effect it has had on the patient, although the full picture will take time to emerge. Ask questions, and write down the answers. You are simply in no condition to take in information properly, so you need to check your version with your informant. And you need help to remember it all.

Tell the patient what is going on. Many people completely forget that the patient is lying there, desperate to know exactly what has happened, and feeling strange effects that he has never read about. 'I thought I was going mad' is a frequent comment from recovered patients. He can probably take in more than you think, even if he cannot speak or seems semi-conscious. Don't add isolation and unnecessary fear to his problems.

Start exploiting other people. Unless the stroke wears off quickly and completely, you are both going to need help. For all you can tell at this stage, that help may be needed for quite a long time. Start roping it in. In the first 'shock' period, many people will be saying: 'Is there anything I can do?', if only to feel better themselves. Probably, there isn't much they can do yet. But don't just say: 'No, thanks'. Train yourself to thank them heartily and say you will let them know just as soon as you have decided what you need. When you do contact them, days or weeks later, and remind them about their offer, they will rarely be able to turn you down. Be aware that offers of help tend to fade away rather fast, when the immediate emergency is over. People forget. Exploit those first offers! An exhausted carer does the patient no good.

Think about money. We are usually taught to feel that it is rather sordid to think about money at times of crisis, but it's nothing of the kind. You may be dealing with one working person who can no longer work – or two of them. Even if both patient and carer are already retired, expenses are going to shoot up. You need all the financial help you are entitled to. You'll find that it is not very much and that you will have to nag for it. You are surrounded by professionals who can give you advice on what to do – or can tell you where to get that advice. For heaven's sake, take advantage of this.

Practical things you can do

FOR THE PATIENT
At the very beginning, you can:

- Just be there, You don't have to talk all the time. Use touch – it is very reassuring. Bring something to do, so you can sit quietly and just be.
- Talk to the patient – even if she is still unconscious or asleep. She may well be able to hear you, and to understand you.
- If she is conscious or on the way, find out if she can understand you. If you think she can't, talk to her anyway in a reassuring – but adult – way. She has lost none of her intelligence. Establish some kind of communication, if only through touch.
- Tell the staff what name she likes to be called, who she is and what her interests are. Also tell them what her personality is like. How does she like to be treated?
- Watch for any changes in her condition. If you notice anything, tell the staff. It could be a change for the better, a change for the worse, unusual (for her) actions.
- Make sure the staff tell the patient about anything they do to her: 'We're going to turn you on to the other side ...' and so on. Talk her through things yourself.
- Make sure she has any aid she always uses: glasses, hearing aid, dentures and so on.
- Tell the staff about any other medical condition you know of.

To help care for the patient, you can:

- Watch what the staff do. Learn how they do things – and why. The first part of Chapter 3 will explain much of it.
- Start helping the staff, so you can get advantage from their personal teaching. Keep asking 'why?'
- Take charge occasionally of a task such as feeding, if the patient needs help with this. You probably have more time than the nurses to do it properly.
- Ask staff to suggest things you can bring in for the patient. Luxury incontinence pads might be more to the point than chocolates.
- Find out about any drugs the patient is being given: what they are, the instructions for taking them, what they are for, and what the side effects might be. Look out for side effects – often a change of drug is well worth making.
- Ask the staff, as soon as anything is known, what the effects of the stroke will be. Show them the list in Section 1 (pages 7–10) and ask them to note down which of them the patient seems to be suffering – and any other effects they have noticed.

As soon as possible (day one, ideally) make sure the patient is brought back into the real world:

- Bring visitors – but make sure they understand how to treat the patient, before they come in. Make sure they don't exhaust the patient.
- Bring in a clock and/or calendar.
- Bring familiar objects, like photographs.
- Bring flowers or leaves.
- Bring pets, if allowed.

- Bring food, if allowed (check this one carefully).
- Bring newspapers and other reminders of what is going on outside.
- As soon as he can be got into a wheelchair, take him outside the building.
- Make sure he has music if he wants it. Check what the hospital radio is playing, and if necessary bring in a radio or cassette player.
- Talk! Even if he doesn't respond, he may well do so next time, or the time after that.

FOR YOURSELF

- Get someone to relieve you at the patient's bedside. Go outdoors. Get a break.
- Get someone to relieve you so you can relax sometimes. Don't exhaust yourself.
- Cry every time you feel like crying. You need to get all these feelings *out*, to stop them building up inside you.
- Contact your employers or the patient's employers, if relevant. Explain that the effects of the stroke cannot be estimated at this stage. Discuss getting time off sick, paid leave, unpaid leave or whatever is appropriate.
- Find out what financial benefits are available, from employers and from the state. Don't put it off. Give the job to somebody else if necessary.
- Promise yourself that you will look after your own needs as well as the patient's. Unless you do, you'll make a bad job of caring.

FOR THE FUTURE

The patient will start to recover quite fast. But this recovery reaches its limit quite soon – within the first two or three weeks, usually.

It may be a complete recovery. Small strokes may not cause permanent, noticeable damage although some brain cells will indeed have died and can't be replaced. Some recoveries take longer, and need active rehabilitation work for quite a long time. To make it as easy and as pleasant as possible, it needs to be planned. This book will show you how.

FOR NOW
As soon as you can think straight, you need to get a clear idea of what needs to be done. With stroke, getting better doesn't happen by chance.

So, the minute the patient regains consciousness, there are certain things that have to be done right – consistently, by everyone involved. These give the patient the maximum chance of making the best possible recovery. They save wear and tear on the carer, too!

Professionals understand this well – doctors, nurses, therapists. Watch what they do, ask questions, jot down notes. Get as much out of them as you can. In the early days the physiotherapist and (if the patient can't communicate) the speech therapist are very important.

Things you need to know

There are just seven absolute essentials you need to know right from the start. They explain why the professionals do the things they do. And they explain what you need to do.

There's a lot of information to take in – and neither patient nor carer is in an ideal state to handle it all! So concentrate on the seven things you must understand and practise:

THE SEVEN ESSENTIALS

Communicating

If the patient can't speak and/or can't understand words, you can (and must) get some kind of communication going right away. See Section 6 – and see a speech therapist.

Immobility

Someone who lies still all the time can get breathing problems. And muscles – even healthy ones – lose their power very quickly if they are not used. Getting some movement is a priority. See page 50.

Pressure areas

If the patient can't move much, constant pressure on one part of the body can cause breakdown of the skin, and very nasty sores. This can happen surprisingly easily, and the sores can go surprisingly deep. See page 48.

Lifting

If the patient can't move much, someone will have to help. If it isn't done properly, it can very easily give the helper a back injury – which can range from painful to downright catastrophic. See page 47.

Shoulder

Paralysed shoulders are very vulnerable. Bad positioning, and bad moving, can cause painful injury and permanent damage. See page 51.

The weak side

Movement and power in the weak side – however small – must be encouraged from the start. There is such a thing as 'learned non-use' so ignoring the weak side will teach it to be more helpless than it need be. What's more, using the strong side in unusual movements 'to compensate' will break down the weak side's ability to recover.

Balanced position

This is the big one. Keeping the two sides of the body in balance is the way to make it recover in a normal way. Without care, one side will tighten up and make arm, leg and trunk twisted. The trick is to keep the whole body in the right position from head to toe, with both sides matching. See page 53.

Both patient and carer need to know these rules, understand how important they are, talk about them (if possible) and encourage each other to remember them. This may not be easy if patient is confused, has problems with perception, does not understand language, or is apathetic and uncooperative. If the patient is in hospital, the nurses should be using the seven essentials in their daily care, guided by the physiotherapist. Watch them to get some tips.

Carrying out the seven essentials may not be easy. But the effort is the best investment you can make towards maximum recovery. The price of neglecting them really can be quite heavy.

Detailed instructions are given in the next section. For the moment just make sure you know *why* the seven essentials are so important. Both of you.

Finally ...

The seven essentials are the really practical things that need to become second nature. Overleaf are a few wider points that are also important. Take them to heart!

Stroke

CARING

- Caring well means getting plenty of help, *before* the need gets desperate. Look at Section 8, *Other people*, and then 9, *Resources*.
- The carer's needs are as important as the patient's: a miserable, exhausted carer is a bad carer.
- Emotional as well as physical needs must be met. Both patient and carer need the freedom to express feelings.
- Don't block the patient away from the real world, whether it's worries about money (she'll be fully aware of these anyway) or simply what the weather's like today.
- Take time, sometimes, to put yourself in your partner's shoes. Use your imagination.
- Money is important. You are entitled to financial help. Ask about it. Get it.

RECOVERY

- Really good early care is the key to final recovery – especially position and balance (see Section 3, *Early days*).
- Rehabilitation starts at once – as soon as the patient regains consciousness.
- Rehabilitation goes on 24 hours a day! Everyone who deals with the patient needs to do things exactly the same way, or they will undo each other's good work.
- Good professional advice, tailored to your particular needs (clearly stated) is very, very useful.
- The patient, and the carer, are the experts on the particular stroke, and the relationship and lifestyle it is happening to. Help the professionals find out how it is for *you*, so they can tailor-make their advice. Tell them about feelings, as well as facts.

HOW NOT TO PANIC

Problems can seem overwhelming: so many of them, so complicated, so upsetting. But there are common sense ways to make things easier to handle.

First – give the problem a name. If something is floating around in the back of your mind, it can be made a lot less powerful if you focus your attention on it and define exactly what it is. It may be awful. It may be comparatively trivial (though not to you). But at least you know what you're up against.

Rather than a great cloud of anxiety, you have got, for example:

1 I'm so afraid that he/she will die.
2 I'm afraid I won't be able to cope.
3 I don't want to have to cope with this.
4 My feet hurt.

Now – think about it and talk about it. What makes this problem so awful? What is it all about in detail? Talking to somebody else is amazingly effective in making your burden lighter (if they don't judge you and don't interrupt with opinions and advice). Somehow, just telling and being heard has the magical effect of 'dumping' the problem. And, when you have seen the problem in all its glory, you will see some possible solutions or next steps that should help you get rid of this problem.

So – carry out these next steps, however small they seem. For example:

1 You can ask a professional what the chances are of your partner dying.
2 You can ask for information on what caring will consist of.

3 You can confide your feelings to a trusted person.
4 You can put your feet up, or make a definite promise to give your feet a specific treat as soon as you can.

Now – evaluate. Did your action solve the problem completely? If so, congratulate yourself and move on to another problem.

Or is there still something niggling? Or are you landed with a whole new set of problems instead of the original one? If so, return to the problem and have another think about it and another talk about it, and try another step.

All this thinking and trying things can seem like hard work. But it is far, far better than being plagued by formless worries. You are doing something, and that will always make you feel better than doing nothing.

CARE PLANNING

In fact, the kind of process outlined above is very like the process used by professionals in planning their own work. Nurses usually call it 'the nursing process', doctors might call it 'problem-oriented medical records', and there are many other names. But they all describe the common sense way of pinning down problems and working at them.

Look at the notes being used by the nurses (either in hospital or in the home). For instance, they will probably list the need to prevent the patient getting pressure sores (see page 30). So – a problem is clearly defined.

Cultivate the habit of defining your problems clearly, and working out solutions in small, easy steps. If you try something and it doesn't work, try something else.

Be encouraging, to yourselves and each other (more about this in Section 4).

PLANNING
- Be precise about problems and solutions. Don't let things overwhelm you.
- Choose which problems to work on first of all: the easiest!
- Find out what you need to deal with them – information? a helper? money?
- Map out your plan of action in small, easy steps. This makes success likely.
- Success is to be built on. Set the next easy goal.
- Failure is to be analysed – everything that doesn't work is a clue to what *would* work.
- Success is to be celebrated!

BEING POSITIVE
- Both patient and carer need to feel valued.
- Feelings have something to tell you. They are not enemies, to be suppressed.
- Look at the good things, as well as the bad. Pay extra attention to them.
- Don't be all or nothing. A small success is still a success.
- Remember that carer and patient are still normal people. Normal people have rows, get fed up, can't be bothered to get dressed occasionally. Normal people have good times, too ...

Workbook no 1

So, your first workbook activity is to apply the care plan approach to whatever is bothering you right now.

1 Find out what the problems are
  Write down everything that bothers you, large and small. What do you want to be able to do, that you

can't do now? Eat without help? Play golf? Whatever!

2 Choose a goal and break it down

Pick on the easiest changes you can make. You may not be able to go water-skiing tomorrow, but you can make a start on washing yourself. Making a start is the vital thing. Choose an easy goal, and break it down into tiny steps. You may not be able to wash your whole body, but how about washing your face?

3 Take the first step

4 See if it worked

The trick is to make your planning more and more precise. Suppose the patient didn't manage to wash his face. Was it because he simply didn't want to? Change the goal. Was it because his weak hand can't manage? Use the strong hand to guide it. Was it because the patient can't sit up and balance well enough? Work on that.

The more precise you can be, the better your plans will work. You need to know *exactly* what you are aiming at. Don't make your goal something vague like 'to be more active'. What does 'more active' mean? How do you know when you've got there? Instead, make the goal something like 'stand up unaided for one minute more, every day'. Then it will be obvious if you've done it or not. The smaller the goal, the more likely is success. Success breeds confidence and the will to succeed at the next step.

A failure is never a waste of time. You've learned something. What led to the failure – the patient was tired? His leg hurt? What? And what can be changed to stop this happening again? Was the original goal unrealistic for some reason you had not thought of?

A success is to be celebrated. You should always stress what the patient *can* do – however small. Not what he can't do.

SEVEN THINKING TIPS

Getting to grips with a problem or solution can be difficult. Here are some ways to start pinning it down.

- Remember that the first step towards planning an action is to *think*.
- When you're not sure *what* you're faced with, scribble down every thought in your head, nice or nasty, important or trivial. Now see if you spot any patterns.
- Give feelings and problems a worry score between 1 and 10. If it's over, say, 7 it's probably a priority. If the score goes up later on, it's certainly a priority.
- When faced with a problem, check that it's *your* problem. If necessary, hand it back to the person who has power to deal with it. Or ask somebody else to solve it for you!
- When making a difficult decision: write a list of the advantages and a list of the disadvantages. Ask – what's the best thing that could happen? What's the worst thing that could happen?
- When change is needed, pick the smallest, easiest thing you can change and *do it*.
- Catch yourself using killer phrases like: 'I'm fine' ... 'Of course I'm all right' ... 'Don't bother' ... 'I can manage'. Are you giving out messages which stop people from helping?

MAKE A START

Think in terms of making *small steps*. Care plans are all about making it easy to get started, and easy to be successful. This, obviously, motivates people to have a go. And if you can be precise about what an action is aiming to achieve, it is easy to tell whether it is doing any good or not.

So start thinking about care planning, and how it can be used. What problems are uppermost in your mind at the moment? Could care planning have anything to help you get to grips with it? Don't panic – do something!

3

EARLY DAYS

This section explains the basics for care in the first few days, whether this takes place at home or in hospital. Many stroke patients never go into hospital at all. Many others are discharged home while still quite highly dependent. Others, again, may have to spend a while at home while they wait for a place in a special rehabilitation unit.

Even in hospital, the carer can help out. She can practise techniques while there are skilled staff around to help and advise. (The physiotherapist, in particular, is a valuable resource who should be called on while you have the chance). At worst, the carer may find she has to supplement the work of the nurses because staffing is short.

Now it's time to master the details of the Seven Essentials. These are given on pages 46 onwards, so take a look. And get ready for the patient's homecoming ...

Being at home

If the doctors think the patient should be at home, this is almost always a very good sign: it means they see no danger to his life, either from the stroke itself or from complications it may cause.

It does *not* mean that there's no further hope of progress. On the contrary, patients are likely to do better in a familiar setting, or with familiar people. It will be easier for them to get back in touch with the world, and to engage in activities which have some meaning. But do please remember that the rapid recovery made in the first two or three weeks, as the brain gets over its injuries, does not continue at the same pace. Once the 'spontaneous' recovery is over, the rest is down to hard work. Try not to be disappointed; try not to expect the earth.

An experienced medical specialist reports that patients who make the quickest and most complete recovery are the ones who are sent home to live alone. They have no choice but to do things for themselves. There's an obvious lesson here, both for patients and for carers. It is possible to do too much for a patient – from the best of motives. It is possible for a patient to be more helpless and demanding than he needs to be – for quite understandable reasons. It can be hard to get the right balance.

For both patient and carer, being at home can be very scary. The responsibilities can seem heavy, no matter how well prepared you thought and hoped you were. Taking care of the seven essentials is a day and night responsibility in itself – never mind all the other things you'll have to be thinking about. Nobody can keep up that kind of workload for long, and nobody should be expected to.

With some people, the 'early days' go on for quite a long time. The paralysis may be severe; disturbance of perception and other mental functions may continue, and give the patient major problems in co-operating; his fear or frustration may create problems all of their own; and both patient and carer will be battling will all kinds of conflicting feelings, about almost everything. You are both likely to get very, very tired.

Get all the help you can

You need extra helpers – anyone you can get – to take over some of the slog. You need them to take on other jobs – from housework to starting the battle to get financial help – so that you are freed to manage the basic care yourself. And remember the word is 'manage' – the carer should be making sure things get done, but not doing absolutely all of them.

You need professional help, too. You need visiting nurses to do some of the work for you. You need nurses, physiotherapists and occupational therapists to advise you on the ins and outs of getting the work done. This book can explain the ground rules, but a little advice from a professional can do wonders in helping you tailor your actions to the particular problems of your home, the patient's condition, your relationship. You may need a speech therapist to work out ways to communicate with a patient who has lost the power of language.

You may well have communication problems on a deeper level. Both of you will almost certainly need a shoulder to cry on. Both of you will be very aware that life has changed drastically and will feel frightened, angry, self-pitying, resentful – and probably guilty about feeling all these things. All of this is to be expected. Anyone would feel the same way. But is hardly an ideal basis to start a programme of hard work, and responsibility, and mutual co-operation. You need emotional support.

Patient and carer will need to be on the same wavelength

about the work that has to be done, and how you are going to cope with it. You will need to negotiate. Where carrying out intimate tasks is concerned, you may need to be quite frank about what the carer is and is not prepared to do, and what the patient is willing to let outsiders do. If the two points of view are not in harmony, you'll have to sort it out – a sympathetic professional is probably the best person to help the negotiations here, and it is certainly part of her job.

You will almost certainly need financial help, too. A stroke is often a financial catastrophe. Patient or carer – or both of them – may have jobs. For the carer, giving up his or her job is not the only option open, but leave of absence will need to be worked out. Meanwhile, having a sick person at home immediately puts up expenses in all kinds of ways, from heating and telephone bills to special equipment. You are unlikely to have money thrown at you. Getting financial help is one of the worst problems for many patients and carers.

This all sounds very pessimistic. Maybe you won't have any of these problems. But it's much better to be aware at the outset that things can be difficult. Don't aim to be strong. Aim to be aware of problems if they arise, and willing to seek out the help you need wherever you can get it.

Planning your home

The early stages are *not* the time to make major alterations to the home. You don't want to splash out money until you know your financial position (present and future). And you simply don't know, at this point, what you might need in the way of lowered work surfaces, widened doorways, ramps and so on. Nobody can yet predict how full a recovery you will manage between you, and therefore nobody can predict whether or not the patient will manage without a wheelchair, will be able to get up steps and reach every part of home and garden more or less unaided.

But these are a few things you must think about right away ...

THE BED
At first, it might be a good idea to make up a bedroom on the ground floor, if you live in a house with stairs.
Advantage: the patient will not be cut off from most of the household's activity.
Disadvantages: the carer will have tiring trips up and down the stairs during the night and if he or she is married to the patient, the separation is very hurtful. The patient may not have easy access to the bathroom and will have to use invalid devices like commodes and washing bowls for longer than necessary.

- The bed itself should ideally *not* be in a corner. There should be access from both sides. A single bed makes access easier, although again the ultimate aim should be for married patients to sleep in the same bed as their spouse, if they did so before the stroke. Don't get rid of the double bed!
- If the patient has to go in a double bed, place his affected side at the edge.
- The bed's height may need to be adjusted. Too high and it is unsafe for the patient; too low and moving the patient puts an extra strain on the carer's back. Best compromise is a height which allows the patient to put both feet flat on the floor, with knees at right angles. Wooden bed legs could be sawn off to lower the bed; to raise it, place it on blocks (hollowed out for safety) or screw-on mini-legs.

- A bed 'cradle' (perhaps a strong cardboard box) is needed to keep the weight of bedclothes off the patient's feet.
- The ideal bed is *not* a divan. This has no space underneath, and the patient will need to put his feet under the bed when learning to sit and stand.
- The ideal mattress is not sagging. A piece of perforated hardboard underneath will help.
- The bed needs some kind of headboard if possible, to help the patient sit up.
- The bed must *not* have a footboard, keeping feet at right angles to the legs. This might seem a good way to stop the patient's feet from pointing or 'dropping', but in practice it has the opposite effect.

THE BEDSIDE

A bedside table is a must. The patient needs access to the things he needs, without having them handed to him. He also needs to be stimulated by interesting objects close at hand.

- First of all, place the table next to the patient's unaffected (good) side. He will have a tendency to slump over towards his affected (weak) side. If he has to stretch out to reach the table, he will automatically start to correct this slump.
- As soon as the patient can balance when sitting up, however, the table should be moved to his affected side. This will probably not be popular with him – but practising using his weak, affected side is useful. More important, he will tend to reach across his body in order to go on using the good arm – which produces several beneficial reactions through the sensory part of the

nervous system. All this will be an extra strain at
first, however, if your patient is simply not aware of
the world on his affected side. Constant reminders will
be needed.

- A table which can slide out over the bed is a good
investment. In the early days, it will be invaluable for
keeping his affected arm straight out in front of him. In
time, it will be a useful work surface which can also be
used across a chair.
- Another worthwhile investment might be a baby alarm
or intercom, to give peace of mind at night to carers
sleeping in another room. It can save effort during the
day, too. The more the carer can leave the patient alone
with a clear conscience, even for a few minutes, the
better. If you can't manage an intercom, try a bell.

Safety
The patient should get out of bed as soon as possible. Both
patient and carer need to be confident she can do so safely.

- Check for sliding mats, polished floors, low tables,
trailing flexes and general clutter. She will have enough
to concentrate on without having to see to her own
safety.
- Make sure fires and heaters are guarded. A fall is always
possible, and need not be a disaster.
- Make sure lighting is good. The patient's vision and
confidence may be poor. Gloomy lighting is depressing,
too.
- Try to make sure heating is adequate. People lose heat
if they cannot move much.
- Remember that the patient may not feel much on her
affected side. Get her into the habit of checking that this

side of her body is not open to damage in any way.
This will be an effort if the patient is not really aware
of that side.

THE CHAIR
Getting the patient out of bed will be a priority. He may
not be ready to walk for some time, but sitting in a chair
should be well within his capacity and will make him feel a
lot more normal and in control. But keep these sessions
quite short at first. If he can't change position easily he will
get uncomfortable and may slip out of that vital balanced
position. So – no more than three hours.

- The chair should be fairly high, so the patient can get
  in and out and the carer's back is safeguarded. Use the
  same rule of thumb as for bed height. If necessary, raise
  the chair on blocks or screw-in extensions.
- A firm cushion placed on the seat can also add useful
  height easily.
- A firm cushion at the back of the chair may also be a
  good idea. Try it out.
- A table which goes across the chair is important – to
  support the affected arm in the right position and to act
  as a surface for activities. A DIY enthusiast friend may
  be able to improvise something.
- Bars between the front legs of the chair should be
  avoided. They prevent the patient putting his feet
  under the chair to get up.

Lifting

People are heavy – and you can't drop them if things take an awkward turn. The main danger is to the lifter's back. Backs are tricky things, and damage may well not be curable. A series of small strains and injuries can build up into permanent pain. In some cases a single mishandled lift can cause real disability. Take your back seriously.

- Ask your physiotherapist for a demonstration of good lifting, and any tips she has for handling this particular patient.
- Keep your back as straight as possible.
- Bend your knees, not your back. Leg muscles are stronger than back muscles. Get your legs to do the actual work of lifting.
- Keep feet fairly wide apart. This makes you more stable, and less likely to be pulled off-balance.
- Keep close to the person you are helping. Lifting at arm's length strains the back; keeping close means you can use your body to help support the patient's weight.
- Place at least one foot in the direction you are moving towards – one foot pointing sideways, for instance, if you're moving to the side. This prevents twisting.
- Make sure the patient knows what you're doing, and can co-operate. Give instructions, count up to lift-off and so on.
- Just before you lift, tuck your chin under. This helps stabilize your spine.
- Until the patient is able to help you a bit, or until you've become fairly skilled at it, try all you can to get someone to help you.

- If you're using just one arm for a small shift of position, place the other one on a firm surface (your knee, if necessary) for extra support.

Pressure sores

People shift around in their seats all the time because they get uncomfortable. But stroke patients may have no feeling on the affected side, and may not be able to move anyway. This means that pressure builds up and is not relieved.

The problem shows up in the tiny blood capillaries, deep in the tissue. They cannot take much pressure, and are squashed flat. This stops the blood flowing through them, which feeds the tissue and keeps it alive. Shifting about means that no capillaries are flattened for too long, so they can keep doing their job. But if you can't shift about, constant pressure keeps a certain group of capillaries flattened for too long and the tissue dies.

You've probably heard of 'skin sores' or 'bed sores'. But they don't just affect the skin, and you don't just get them in bed. Immobility in bed, chair or wheelchair can all lead to sores – pressure sores is a better name for them. They can start at skin level and work their way down, or they can start deep in the tissue and reveal themselves only when they've worked their way up to the surface. Bad sores are dreadful – you can put your fist into them. And they can start quite easily. Prevention is very much better than cure (although it's not always possible in very ill patients).

- Make sure the patient changes position regularly – day and night. He will do this naturally once his paralysis starts to wear off but in the meantime there's no substitute for moving him yourself. If he is very

Pressure sores – what's the risk?

Everyone needs to be careful about pressure sores, if full movement is not possible. There is no exception to this rule. All the same, some people are at *extra* risk. This score system was devised by Doreen Norton, a British nurse, to pinpoint patients who need *scrupulous attention*. Ask a professional to help you fill it in, if necessary. Simply look at each column in turn and choose the description which fits the patient best. Put a ring round the number which goes with it. Then add up all the numbers.

Physical Condition		Mental Condition		Activity		Mobility		Incontinence	
Good	4	Alert	4	Walking	4	Complete	4	None	4
Fair	3	Apathetic	3	Walks with help	3	Slightly limited	3	Occasional	3
Poor	2	Confused	2	Chair-bound	2	Very limited	2	Usually urine	2
Very bad	1	Stupor	1	Bed-bound	1	Immobile	1	Double (urine & faeces)	1

If you score 14 or less, special care is needed.

vulnerable, you may need to do this every two hours. Take professional advice, and calculate the risk with our chart.

- Get to know the areas where pressure falls hardest. If the patient is on his side (by far the best position for stroke patients) these are: ankles, knees, hips, elbows, shoulders, side of head. If he's on his back, or in a chair, add: heels, toes, base of spine, buttocks. Check that

pressure here gets relieved, and look out for danger signs
– skin which is red, dry or broken. Get advice at once.

* Lie the patient on a sheepskin, which spreads out the
pressure.
* If paralysis persists, you may need a special mattress (on
hire or loan). There are various kinds, all designed to
vary the pressure and reduce the need for moving.
* Look out for extra sources of pressure, like hard objects
lost in the bed. Even crumbs, or wrinkles in the sheets,
can put extra pressure on skin.
* Try to lift the patient – not drag him along. Friction can
make skin break down.
* Don't rub the skin at pressure areas – friction again.
* If the patient is incontinent, don't let him lie in wet
sheets. This damages skin too.
* Look out for accidental pressure – an arm lying against a
hard object, and so on. The patient may not notice he is
causing pressure in this way and will need to learn to
look out.

Immobility

Astronauts have to keep moving and exercising in space, or
their muscles are badly weakened and their bones lose calcium. Stroke patients are no different – except that their
powers of recovery are rather less.

Unless a professional tells you otherwise, there is no reason not to get the patient out of bed straightaway (but be
careful with lifting!). It's psychologically healthy to get back
to normal as soon as possible, too. But remember – not for
too long.

There is no reason for a stroke patient to rest constantly
(unless he has some other trouble, such as a recent heart

attack, and you have been advised accordingly). On the contrary, it is good for both patient and carer to encourage every possible activity.

- Be sensitive to any special sensory losses which may affect the patient's confidence or mobility. Make sure you know just what the problems are – get the professionals to fill in the checklist (pages 7–10) for you.
- Look at the **Weak side** section overleaf for special advice on some of these.

Shoulder care

There is a tendency for a paralysed shoulder to droop downwards. Unfortunately, this can cause a lot of damage. The arm has to move in so many directions that the shoulder joint is quite unstable and liable to dislocate if its supporting muscles are weak.

This is more or less what happens if the shoulder is allowed to droop. This is very painful and may take a very long time to get better.

- Never pull the arm or shoulder.
- Never place your hand in the patient's armpit on the weak side (to lift him, for instance).
- Stick to the rules in the **General position** section, and pay special attention to the shoulder when positioning the patient.
- The patient needs to take over control of his own positioning as soon as possible. It may be an incentive if he knows that pain could be the penalty for ignoring it!
- The physiotherapist may prescribe a cuff going round the upper arm, to keep the shoulder in place.

The weak side

A great deal is being learned about the nervous system's power to recover. There is evidence that it can 're-learn' powers which, years ago, would have been thought to be lost for good.

The nervous system learns partly by experience. The way the patient moves (or is moved) dictates how he will move in the future. That's why general position is so important. The bad news is that under-use can train the nervous system to *lose* function. The result is called 'learned non-use', and it makes it all the harder to rehabilitate an affected arm or leg.

- Try hard not to use the 'good' side – frustrating though this is, it will lead to better all-round recovery in the end.
- Place interesting objects – from bedside tables to visitors! – on the affected side, so the patient uses it as much as possible.
- Speak to the patient from his affected side.
- Make special efforts with patients who simply take no notice of the affected side and feel it doesn't belong to them (anosognosia). It may be a long learning process.
- Give extra encouragement, too, to patients who can't see on the affected side.
- Don't expect any of this to be easy. If you have a 'good' and a 'bad' side, you will naturally want to use the good side because it is so much easier. Anger or tears will, equally naturally, result from the effort of using the bad side.

General position

Many people have a vision of the 'typical stroke patient' – head on one side, arm bent across the body, fingers stuck in a claw-like grip, leg dragging, foot dragging. That's exactly what used to happen in the bad old days – and could still happen.

Luckily treatment has been revolutionized in recent years, largely through the ideas of a physiotherapist called Berta Bobath. We have the power to prevent all that deformity. How? From the very start – even if the patient is unconscious – she has to be placed in the right position.

Immediately after the stroke, the affected limbs are floppy (flaccid). The brain is not properly in control of

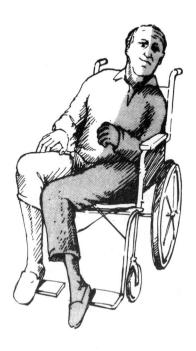

them. All muscles, at all times, have a certain degree of 'tone'. Even when they are resting, they are pulled up tight to some extent, especially the muscles which counter the downward pull of gravity.

When the brain is no longer properly in charge, after a stroke, the anti-gravity muscles become more dominant than they should be. The limbs are pulled into tightened 'typical stroke patient' positions (sometimes called 'spasticity').

If they are allowed to stay like that, the muscles become permanently shortened and can no longer stretch out again. By the time the patient has recovered some control and power in her affected limbs, it is too late. And the patient is very much more disabled than she need have been.

Another important concept is balance, throughout the whole body. The patient needs to develop the ability to balance on her own, instead of slumping over towards her affected side. If she is propped up on that side, the imbalance is encouraged and the affected side is not trained to balance things up for itself.

Good balance is the foundation for sitting, standing and walking – as you'll know if you've watched a baby learning to do these things. Good balance also helps the whole nervous system to recover. It learns partly from experience, and can get into bad habits like any other body system.

As with the rules for arm and leg, some patients will find it particularly difficult to pay attention to their affected side. A mirror will help, and so will constant reminders, and tricks like always placing yourself on the affected (weak) side.

Until the patient regains strength and balance, her position will have to be checked at least every two or three hours, day and night. As soon as possible, she should get into the habit of checking for herself that she has:

- neck and spine straight
- shoulders level
- both elbows, wrists, and shoulders straight – supported in front of her, not hanging down
- leg in line with the body
- foot at right angles to leg – not 'dropped'
- in short – both sides level and the same, from head to toe

It's uncomfortable to be stuck in the same position for more than two or three hours – and, of course, there's the danger of pressure sores. So even a good position has to be changed to another good position regularly. When she's lying down, it's a question of turning her from one side to the other. Lying on the side is the best possible position for avoiding spasticity (tightened muscles).

Lying, turning and moving all have to be done the right way – right from the start. It will save both of you endless problems and is worth every effort. Turn to page 62 for advice, and follow it.

Tiresome tasks

In the early days, a stroke patient may need help with all kinds of activities he would normally do for himself, and with irritating weaknesses he would rather not have. This is rather humiliating, and both patient and carer may well dislike and resent what they have to do.

Carers may get over some of their inhibitions by pretending to themselves that they are nurses when they carry out these routines. It sounds silly, but it can be quite effective in helping to maintain a normal relationship with the patient when you are *not* carrying out these tasks.

Patients (and carers!) need to understand that most of these problems will wear off, often quite soon. The aim must be to return the patient to independence as soon as possible. Carers must steel themselves to give only the help which is absolutely necessary, and keep up the patient's self-esteem.

INCONTINENCE

It is not uncommon for stroke patients to lose control of bladder, and possibly bowels, in the first few days. This nearly always rights itself quite soon, usually when the patient can get out of bed (another reason for encouraging mobility!). In the meantime:

- Don't cut down on liquids, except perhaps last thing at night. Dehydration is very bad for anyone. What's more, the urine will become more concentrated, which brings a risk of infection and actually encourages incontinence.
- Don't let the patient lie in wet or soiled clothes or sheets. It's humiliating and can lead to pressure sores.
- Don't forget that patients who can't speak need some way to express their needs.
- Guard against constipation, with high fibre foods and plenty of liquid. Constipation can be unhealthy and uncomfortable, and one of its stranger effects is to encourage diarrhoea to flow around faeces which have hardened in the rectum.
- You can buy attractive pants (male or female) which hold an absorbent pad and direct moisture away from the body – the effect of a nappy without the looks.
- Cheap incontinence pads are a false economy. Go for size, comfort and absorbency.

- You can buy or borrow a light plastic (male or female) urinal to use in bed.
- There are other possibilities if problems persist. A nurse or continence adviser can produce a sheath to go over the penis, or even a tiny tube (catheter) which goes into the bladder and feeds into a bag.
- If you notice that urine is dark, or smells, report it. There may be an infection.

In some patients, incontinence won't go away after a few days. It is quite a common problem even in perfectly healthy people, especially as they get older. Quite a lot, however, can be done to help. People have at last realized that incontinence is a matter for specialists, usually called continence advisers. It is very well worth seeking one out. Incontinence, and the work it can cause if it isn't dealt with, is a miserable problem. Don't assume that you just have to live with it. Get help.

SWALLOWING

Inability to swallow (dysphagia) affects about a third of early stroke patients. This can be, at best, messy and, at worst, very frightening. The problem, oddly enough, is usually worse with liquids than with solids. Advice from a nurse or speech therapist, and if possible a dietitian, is vital. If the patient is not in hospital, ask your doctor to refer you for advice.

- If you suspect dysphagia, the only liquid used should be plain water (which can't do much harm if a little goes into the lungs by mistake). If it won't go down, don't persist.
- Make sure the patient doesn't become dehydrated, however.

- The easiest texture to swallow is a thickened, smooth liquid.
- Small mouthfuls are best — use a teaspoon or straw to help control intake. Place it in the non-affected side of the mouth.
- Sucking a jelly cube (check the patient *can* suck) is another way to introduce liquid.
- Avoid food with 'bits' in it, like soup with vegetables. This is the hardest of all to swallow.
- Sitting upright is the best posture.
- After the meal, check that no food is left in the mouth. It could lead to choking or an embarrassing spill-out later on.
- Review progress, with expert advice. You don't want to be stuck with things like straws and baby-style food for any longer than necessary.
- If serious problems persist, a feeding tube through the nose may be preferable to long, miserable struggles which exhaust the patient and make it hard to eat a good diet.

DRIBBLING
Weakened facial muscles can lead to this embarrassing tendency. Most patients will be keen to control it, if they know how. What happens is that saliva pools in the cheek on the affected side of the face. The patient can't feel it is there, and can't stop it leaking out. The answer is to learn a few habits:

- Try to keep swallowing regularly.
- Don't bend the head forward — it's asking for trouble.
- Keep lips closed. Pursing them round a small stick or straw is good practice, and helps you to remember when you're concentrating on something else.

- Keep a handkerchief or tissue handy!
- Practise facial exercises (use a mirror) to strengthen muscles. A speech therapist can suggest some, which are likely to include: open and close mouth, smile, purse lips, say 'oo' and 'ee', move tongue from corner to corner of the mouth, stick tongue out and bend its tip up and down, run tongue round the inside of the mouth.

Daily living

So far, this section has been all about hard work and using technical knowledge. This is how it has to be, and you can be assured that maximum effort on these early problems really will lead to maximum recovery quite soon.

There are two things to remember. First, most patients get tired very easily. This is hardly surprising, as the simplest activities – like moving and speaking – have suddenly become both physically and mentally demanding. The sheer frustration of having to work so hard at such simple things is exhausting in itself. (Carers probably feel much the same!) Both of you, then, need to plan in periods of peace and quiet. Both of you probably need to get away from each other for some part of the day.

Second, and closely related, is the question of morale and motivation. It is not particularly exciting having to carry out endless 'drills' for everything from how you sit to how you eat. Nor do the basic tasks of the early days make the patient seem exciting or attractive, or the carer admiring and sympathetic. Both are, probably, still appalled by what has happened. Both are aware that things have changed, and they don't feel good about it.

There will be a lot of emotional sorting out to do. There will be a lot of battles over who does what, and how independent the patient is willing to be. In between all the tasks, you'll need to start getting to grips with this.

One thing will help a lot: getting back as soon as possible to daily living. Small pleasures, small activities, will count for much. They will also give both of you a chance to make contact in more satisfying ways and – importantly – a chance to use your own ingenuity to solve problems. The first few days are not too soon to start working on the **Daily living** section (page 168).

GROOMING

Patients need to look their best, and carers need to see them looking their best. From day one, pay attention to:

- Shaving (an electric razor is much easier).
- Hair (perhaps a hairdresser can visit at first, although you should aim to go out as soon as possible. Meanwhile the patient can brush and comb).
- Make-up (the carer can apply it at first – but must not make a habit of it).
- Personal hygiene (washing is fairly easy to manage without any special advice, and perfume or aftershave are an extra pleasure).

It is particularly demoralizing to be 'groomed' by someone else, like a baby. Patients should be well motivated to start taking over some of these tasks themselves. Don't forget to have a mirror handy. Many patients will be afraid their appearance has changed, and in any case a mirror is interesting to look at. Washing and making up are very useful for patients who are not aware of their affected side. Watch and remind them to do both sides.

The affected hand should not be left out as the patient starts to take care of his own appearance. He can hold the relevant object in his weak hand and use the strong one to guide it.

DRESSING

As soon as the patient can get out of bed (and that should be as soon as possible), he or she should be in 'normal' clothes as far as possible. This is probably less of a problem for women, who can look and feel normal in an attractive house-coat or a bright tracksuit. Some men may feel rather more conservative about things. But the more casual parts of their wardrobes should yield something that's easy to wear. Garments with elasticated waists or front fastenings are easiest.

Getting dressed is a long and complicated task, so it won't be mastered in the first few days. But some finishing touches can be left for the patient to do right from the start – choosing jewellery or a scarf, arranging a necktie, pulling down sleeves and so on.

This is how to dress someone with an affected arm or leg:

- Put the weak arm into the sleeve first. This leaves more room for manoeuvre (remember to take great care with the shoulder). When undressing, take out the stronger arm first.
- For trousers, lie down, bend the weak leg and put the trouser leg on it. Straighten the leg and pull up the trouser leg as far as possible. Then do the same with the stronger leg. Now pull the trousers all the way up by rocking from hip to hip. Once the patient can sit up, the same basic method can be used – but be sure he is able to keep his balance when sitting, before moving on to this.
- For shoes and socks, it is safest to sit in a chair (with arm rests, and of the right height – a high chair makes

it hard to reach the feet, a low chair makes it hard to bend forward at all). A footstool helps and so does a long-handled shoe horn.

The patient almost certainly needs help in leaning forward, at least in the first few days. The unaffected foot should pose no great problems; the weak foot is the tricky one. Feet are often swollen in the first few days, so take laces out of lace-up shoes, split shoe seams or stick to thick socks or well-fitting slippers. Sloppy slippers are demoralizing – and dangerous.

- A large mirror adds interest and incentive. For people having problems recognizing their affected side, it is very useful indeed.

LYING ON THE AFFECTED SIDE

- Gently pull the affected arm out straight so the shoulder blade moves forward and she is not lying on the point of her shoulder. Don't pull too hard or too far.
- Place her affected thigh in line with the trunk.
- Hold the ankle to bend the knee.
- Bring the good leg forward, bend the knee and put it on a pillow. This is for comfort, pressure area care and to stop her rolling on to her back.
- Make sure the head is not pushed back. This can make the throat uncomfortably tight.
- Use no more than two pillows for the head, to keep the neck straight.
- Try to avoid using cushions behind the patient's back to keep her in position – instinctively, she will push against them. She'll also get very hot.
- A cushion in front of the stomach may be useful to stop her rolling forward.

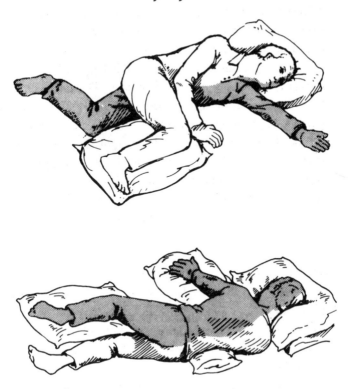

LYING ON THE UNAFFECTED SIDE
- Take the affected arm (the one on top), gently pull it forward and put it on a pillow, elbow straight.
- Keep the weak hip straight, but bend the knee a little and put it on a pillow. This stops her rolling on to her back.
- If necessary, put a small pillow or folded towel under the waist, to keep the spine straight. But remember what's been said about using cushions in **Lying on the affected side.**

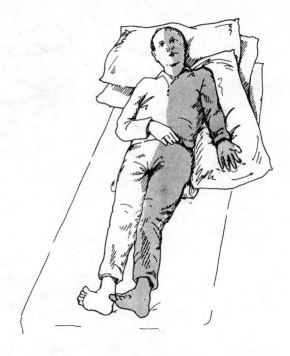

LYING ON THE BACK

This is *not* the best position for keeping the body balanced, and stopping one side from twisting over. But you'll need to use it sometimes when washing, making the bed or giving a bedpan.

- Keep two pillows under the head and bend it slightly towards the good shoulder. Be gentle. Better still, use a foam wedge, or make a wedge from three pillows.
- Put a small pillow or folded towel under the affected hip, just beneath the buttock. This lifts the pelvis forward, relaxes the leg and stops it turning out at the hip. When the patient can balance better, an alternative is to bend both knees, with feet flat on the bed.

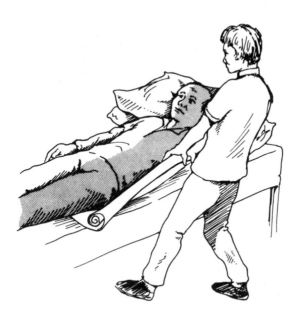

• Straighten the affected arm and put it on a pillow. Make sure fingers and thumb are straight and separated.

CHANGING POSITIONS
To change the side the patient is lying on, you have to roll him over. Your best aid is a folded sheet across the bed, underneath him. By pulling on this, you can move him nearer the edge of the bed so he rolls towards the middle and is in no danger of falling off.

• Roll the patient on to his back (you don't need all the pillow drill because he'll be moving on in a moment).

- Untuck the sheet on both sides.
- On the side you want to move him towards, roll the sheet into a tube.
- Grasp the rolled up sheet and pull, stepping backwards and leaning over the back foot.
- Remember the rules for safe lifting – back straight, knees bent, feet apart.
- Keep arms straight – it's less of a strain.
- If the patient is very heavy, move head and shoulders first, then legs, then hips.

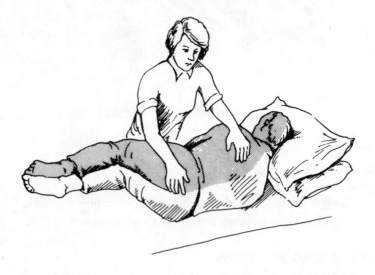

Now you are ready for a safe roll over onto the side, going towards the middle of the bed. Move to the other side of the bed.

- Take the leg furthest from you and cross it over the nearer one.
- Place one hand behind the hip furthest away.

- Place the other hand behind his affected shoulder.
- Pull with both hands together.
- Remember the rules for safe lifting – back straight, knees bent, feet apart.
- Get the patient to help you as soon as he is able to. It is not a difficult movement to make.

SITTING UP

Most stroke patients should be able to sit up in bed, at least part of the time, from very early on. This is good for morale and helps prevent chest infections.

Getting a patient into a sitting position means coping with a lot of his weight. Until he can give you some help, you MUST have a helper for this move. Until he can keep his body in balance by himself, he does need support on his weak side.

- Stand at the affected side, with the helper on the other side.
- Place your arm (the one nearest the head of the bed) across his shoulders at the back. Get the helper to do the same.
- NEVER put your arm in his armpit on the affected side. That shoulder is very vulnerable. Put your arm round his shoulder, on the outside.
- Remember the rules of safe lifting – back straight, knees bent, feet apart.
- Both together, pull the patient up and forward.
- Encourage him to put his chin to his chest – use your free hand to help him if necessary.
- Both you and the helper now turn in towards the bed, so your shoulders can brace the patient's from behind.
- Now he is stable, place the arm you've been using across his back and grasp his waistband (if any) and the hip

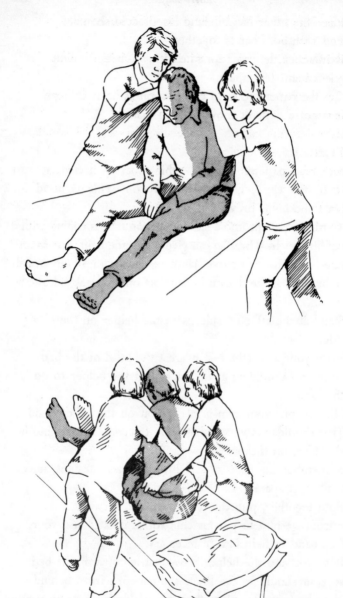

bone beneath it. Your helper does the same, so your arms cross.

- Slide your free arm under his hip. Your helper does the same.
- Now you're ready to lift – back straight, knees bent, feet apart.
- Make sure the patient stays leaning forward. This makes the move much easier.
- Both lift at the same time – count one, two, three, LIFT. Use your legs to do the lifting – not your back. Get the patient to help, too.

When the patient is able to help a bit more, the carer can manage without a helper. But do make sure he has some balance, and knows what he is supposed to be doing and when. Sudden lurches and moves can injure the carer's back.

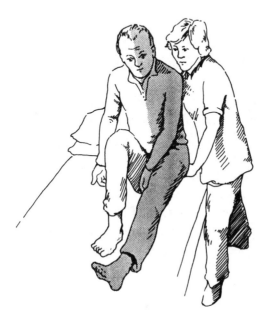

- Get the patient to sit well forward.
- Have his good hand on the bed, slightly behind his body. Keep it relaxed. If he leans on it, it is over-using the good side and endangering that vital body balance.
- Bend his good knee and have the foot flat on the bed.
- Remember the rules of safe lifting – back straight, knees bent, feet apart.
- Count, so you both move together. On the word 'LIFT' the patient pushes to help you.
- It is easier for the patient to press backwards against your shoulder if you are pressing forward against him.

SITTING POSITION

Now the patient has sat up, he needs to be well positioned. Arrange four pillows, as shown, to support him. Pillow number 3 goes behind the patient's affected shoulder to keep it forward. Pillow 4 goes behind his head.

- Get the patient to sit as upright as possible.
- Put a rolled towel under the affected thigh, from buttock to knee. This relaxes the leg and stops it turning out at the hip.
- Put the affected arm – elbow straight, thumb and fingers straight and separated – on a pile of pillows, or a pillow on top of a bed table.

Remember, always, that keeping the two sides of the body in balance is absolutely vital. Take advice from the physiotherapist at every little stage of progress. Until he can do one thing (first lying, then sitting) in a balanced way, you will do no good by moving on to the next stage.

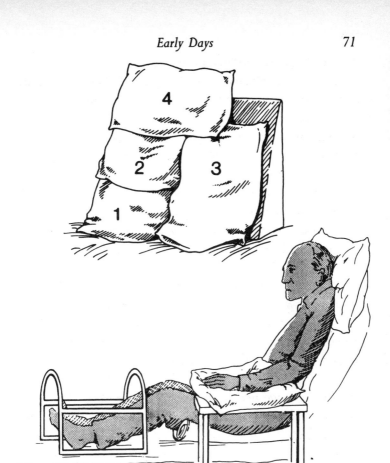

Ready for more ...

So much for the basics of good positioning. And very important they are, to make sure the patient does not end up with a degree of handicap he need never have suffered.

But progress depends on positive work to restore movement and balance. It's time to recap and make sure you both understand this very important principle ...

USING THE AFFECTED SIDE

Most people think that, if a stroke disables one side of the body, the remedy is obvious — make use of the good side. This is just what was done in the bad old days. (And, to be honest, there are still people around who ought to know better — but don't.)

New methods take quite the opposite tack. And the results are much, much more successful. The affected side needs to work much harder, and not be ignored at all. If it is used, it will recover much more of its function.

The strong side, on the other hand, needs to be used in a normal way, in balance with the other side. The patient is not learning a new, distorted way to move. He is re-learning how to move in a normal, balanced way. So ...

- **Don't** prop up the patient when he slumps over towards his weak side. He has to learn to balance by himself. Propping him up just makes the imbalance worse.

- **Do** encourage him to use his weak side as much as possible, right from the start. Nearly every patient has some power in the weak side, and that power must be built on. In the early days, get the patient to use his good hand to hold and guide the weak hand, so it is used as much as possible.

- **Do** persist with the extra effort that will have to be made with patients who can't see the weak side, can't feel it or simply don't know it is there. Remind them. Approach them on the weak side. Talk to them from the weak side. Touch the weak side. Rub it. Hold the weak hand and straighten the fingers gently. Encourage visitors to do the same. It is one of the most useful things they can do to help.

- **Don't** let anyone use an old-fashioned idea which has

become part of the folklore of stroke – making the patient grip or roll a ball or rolled bandage with the weak hand. This is one exercise for the weak side which does *not* have a beneficial effect. It encourages the hand to curl up and stiffen permanently in that position.

- **Do** get the patient to do the following exercises. They can all be done lying down, and they will encourage balance and build up skills for further activities.
- All this will be a big strain on the patient – and the carer! It is bad enough for the patient to 'lose' half his body. Being prevented from using the part that works is ten times more frustrating. Make sure you both realize how worthwhile the results will be. If the patient has no language, get help from a speech therapist.

BED EXERCISES

These bed exercises are a start towards greater independence. And they should begin right away – day one, if at all possible. Patients who are not aware of their affected side will need special help and encouragement.

1 Bridging

If you're using a bedpan, this exercise will prove its worth in making the job easier. But it's really to encourage weight-bearing – the more he pushes down with his feet, the higher the patient can raise his hips. Encourage with a push at the small of the back. If necessary for bedpan purposes, two helpers can stand on opposite sides of the bed and link hands beneath the patient to lift him. As with all lifts, remember – back straight, knees bent, feet apart.

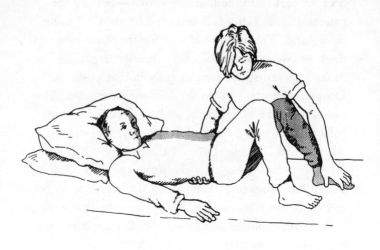

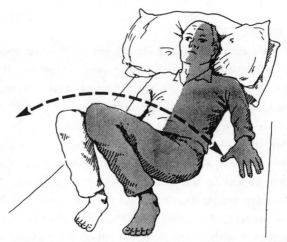

2 Knee swings

Swing knees slowly from side to side as shown. It's important, in particular, to swing as far over as possible towards the good side. This stretches the muscles on the weak side, which are in danger of tightening into spasticity.

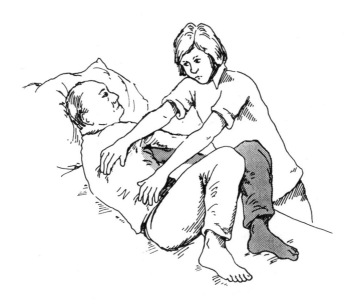

3 Rolling

This, obviously, prepares the patient to help the carer to turn him, and then to do it himself. The sooner this happens, the better. The exercise is an extension of Knee swings, ending up with the patient on his side.

The carer can help by standing at the bedside to reassure him he can't roll right off. If necessary, help pull him over with a hand at shoulder and hip. The patient should watch his hands throughout, to help him turn his head. He should aim to end up with the leg which is on top slightly forward of the other one.

SITTING ON THE BED

Master this, and you are very close to sitting on the bed, and then out of bed in a chair. Many patients can do this as early as the second day – for short periods, at least. Many people, of course, take longer to get this far. The point is that there is every reason to aim at early progress. As soon as possible, both patient and carer need to emphasize what the patient can do, not the functions he has lost. Getting out of bed is an important psychological step.

- Get the patient rolled near the side of the bed, with the carer's help if necessary.
- He should be lying on his affected side, so choose the appropriate side of the bed.
- Lift both feet over the edge of the bed.
- Put one hand (the one nearest the head of the bed) behind the affected shoulder and the other at the back of his knee.
- **Don't** put your hand in his armpit. The affected shoulder is very vulnerable.
- Push upwards with the shoulder hand, and at the same time pull forward with the knee hand. This gets the patient sitting up, legs over the side of the bed.
- Feet should be flat on the floor. If necessary, move nearer the side of the bed.
- To do this, stand close to the patient, feet on either side of the patient's feet.
- Place your arms around the patient's shoulders – this stops the affected shoulder slipping out of place.
- Place your hands under his buttocks.
- If he can't balance yet, get him to put his hands on your waist – *not* round your neck, which could injure you both.
- Rock him to the right (he should be able to help).

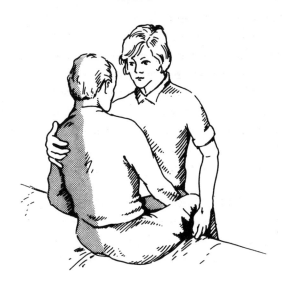

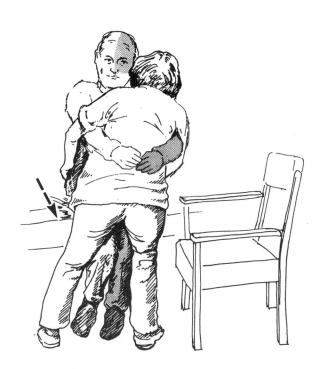

- This takes the weight off the left buttock, so you can pull the leg forward.
- Now do the same thing on the other side.
- Continue until the patient gets to the right place.
- Soon enough, the patient should be able to do this moving unaided. It is a useful way for him to move up and down the bed, and is also the basic technique for putting on trousers.

DO-IT-YOURSELF SITTING

From assisted sitting, it is a short step to independent sitting. Again, the more the patient can take over from the carer the better – for both of them. But at first, the carer will probably need to stand close by, to give the patient confidence.

- Roll on to the affected side, as shown before.
- Bring the good arm across the body and put the hand flat on the bed in front of you.

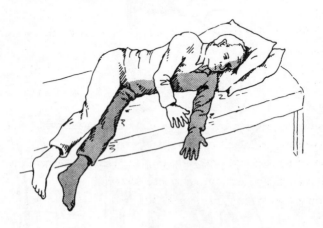

- Push down on this hand so you rise up and can lean on the affected arm.
- Use the good leg to push the affected leg along with it over the side of the bed, and at the same time push down on the hand again. The result should be a sitting position.
- If necessary, rock to get nearer the edge of the bed, as shown before.

MOVING FROM BED TO CHAIR

Now you will need a chair. Make sure you have the right kind of chair, using the checklist on page 46. Now place it close to the bed, and at right angles to it, as near to the head of the bed as possible. Now ...

- Get the patient to the edge of the bed, feet apart and pushed back under the bed.
- Get him to put his arms around your waist.
- Lean well forward.
- Bend your knees.
- Put both hands under his buttocks, or as far down his body as possible.
- Pull him well forward over your shoulder (whichever shoulder you choose).
- Lean back. This will pull the patient clear of the bed.
- Pull him close to you, pressing your knees against his.
- Pivot him round until he has his back to the chair.
- Slowly release the pressure of your knees against his, but make sure he is still bending well forward.
- The patient should now sink into the chair, well back in the seat. If not, he can rock into place.
- If things go wrong, turn to **What if he falls?** on page 126!

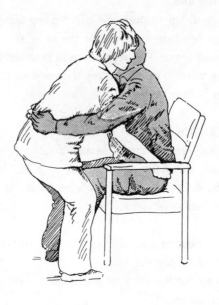

Use the same method to get from chair to commode, and from chair back to bed. The trick is to place the two seats, whatever they are, close to each other and at right angles. Try to get the patient as close to the head of the bed as possible, when you're moving from chair to bed, to save you both the trouble of moving him up the bed.

SITTING POSITION

This is much the same as for sitting up in bed, but with fewer pillows needed! As before, the important pillow is the one which goes behind the affected shoulder (*not* the other side of the body) to keep the shoulder forward. Another pillow will be needed for the head, if the back of the chair does not come high enough. The arm must be positioned as

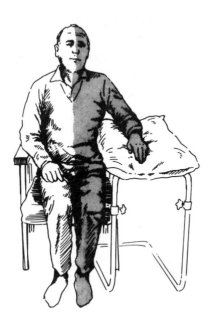

before, using whatever combination of table and pillows works best. Don't just rely on the arm rest of the chair to support the affected (weak) arm. It can easily slip off – damaging the balance, and the arm/shoulder itself.

Finally, remember that pressure sores can happen in a chair, not just in bed. Encourage the patient to raise himself slightly from the chair, say, every half hour at least. And take advice on proper cushioning. Some patients can't keep the affected foot flat on the floor. A rolled towel under the buttock on that side will stop the foot rolling outwards. Remember, don't keep him in the chair for more than about three hours at first.

LOOKING AHEAD

If you have got as far as sitting in a chair you have done really well. Congratulations to both of you! However, the sooner you move on, the better. Tough, but true. Section 5, on *Movement,* outlines the next steps. Some of them you could (and if possible should) be doing from day one ...

Small pleasures

It is very important to prove to the patient (and carer!) that life is still worth living. At first, the patient is very likely to feel disoriented and confused. Many people report that it was months before they really felt human again. So activities need to be undemanding, allowing the patient to appreciate and join in at his own pace. Carers please note: the more you can give the patient to enjoy, the more chance you get to slip away and enjoy something yourself!

Most useful in the early days is the list of small pleasures on pages 156 and 157. They are all things which can get through to a patient who can't communicate. Even if your patient can do so, he will find the suggested activities easy and not too tiring. After all the hard work you have had to do, the last thing you need is leisure activities which are hard work, too!

RECOVERY – THE BASICS

* Rehabilitation starts at once, as soon as the patient regains consciousness.
* Never do anything the patient can do for himself (except perhaps as a special treat).
* Practise little and often. Don't push when either patient or carer is tired.
* Expect hard work. Expect frustration.

- Pick up on every sign of progress, however small. Making a big fuss about something good is a lot more adult than making a big fuss about something bad.
- Self-esteem and confidence are the secrets of rehabilitation.
- Always look ahead. Keep things going ready for the future (e.g. social contacts).

Workbook 2

This whole section is a workbook! Go back through it and look at all the checklists. Go through each one, noting down which things you have to do.

- Write a list
- Choose the most urgent ones.
- Get on with them.
- Choose the easiest ones – whatever they are.
- Do them, too.
- If something doesn't work out, think about *why*.
- That's elementary care planning and action ...

Also, write down as many small pleasures as you, the carer, can get most easily at the moment. Reading? A bath? A quick walk? Music? Write down as many as you can think of – at least 20 – and make sure you actually get round to doing them.

As usual, choose the easiest!

4

FEELINGS

This section centres on the patient, and the carer who is closest to her or him. In particular, it focuses on their feelings. There will be plenty of feelings flying about – violent ones, warm ones, conflicting ones, painful ones, pleasurable ones, feelings which are too awful even to acknowledge, feelings which are too overwhelming to escape.

Patient and carer will have their own private feelings which they try to keep to themselves. Between them, they will also create emotions which can be surprising and frightening. Whatever the relationship was between patient and carer in the past, the stroke will change it.

People don't like change – even change for the better. The unknown is harder to deal with than the familiar. Even a minor stroke, which wears off quickly and completely, is very scary and demands a change of lifestyle, to make sure there are no further strokes. A more severe stroke, of course, changes lifestyle instantly, and totally against your will. Nobody is going to like that.

Of course you'll have feelings about all this. Most cultures, eastern and western, tend to discourage us from expressing or examining our feelings. This means we have very little practice in dealing with them. And this, in turn, puts us very much at their mercy.

But it goes a lot further than that. Any therapist will tell you that morale has much more bearing on the progress achieved than the severity of the handicap. Getting over a stroke can be hard work, both for the patient and the carer. If they can communicate, support each other and comfort each other it will be much easier to get on with the job.

So it's well worth getting in touch with your feelings, acknowledging them and learning how to get something positive out of them. The first feeling you are likely to get is ...

Grief

You have probably already felt the sense of shock described in Section 1. This is very normal, and it's known to be the first stage of something known as the bereavement process, or the grieving process.

This is a pattern which comes up again and again in people who have lost something which is important to them. What is lost may be another person, or it may be a part of oneself, or it may be a certain way of life. People grieve for someone who dies, and they grieve for lost potential (the parents of a handicapped child will grieve for the normal child they expected to have). People grieve for a part of the body if it has been cut off, or a bodily function they have lost.

With stroke, both these types of grieving take place. The stroke patient is not dead, but he is not the person he was before the stroke. He may never be that person again. That person has been lost, and must be mourned, both by the patient himself and by those close to him. Important bodily functions have been lost, too, and with them have gone dignity, motivation, independence.

Many other things have been lost – cherished plans and hopes, a familiar way of life, a relationship which had settled into an accepted groove and – almost certainly – financial security. This is a lot of loss to suffer all at once. No wonder you go into shock.

What happens next also tends to be common to all people who have something to grieve for. It's called denial. This is sheer inability to believe what has happened. It's seen, for instance, in the widow who just can't stop expecting to see her husband around every street corner. With stroke, patient and carer may have expectations which are just as unrealistic.

Some stroke patients have special problems accepting the reality of the stroke, because that's the way their brain damage has taken them. There are patients who insist they are fit to drive, although they can't even see half of the road. There are patients who keep trying to leap to their feet, never learning from experience despite the fact that they fall flat on their faces, every single time.

The next common stage in grieving is anger – the 'why me?' feeling. This goes deeper than the bursts of anger which both patient and carer express when they come up against a day-to-day frustration. There will be plenty of that kind of anger about. But the anger of grieving is much more than that. It is the expression of profound pain and profound disillusionment – a kind of deep hatred of God, humanity or whatever it is you happen to believe in. This, in itself, can be frightening.

When the patient is going through this stage, he is likely to be far more irritable than normal – looking for a scapegoat, perhaps. This is a time when the carer has to clench her teeth and tell herself over and over again: 'It's not *me* he's angry with …' Outside support is invaluable, in the form of a friend, relative or professional who can help the

carer to unload her feelings of being unfairly criticized an
unjustly got at.

Often either patient or carer will mix in a sort of bar-
gaining with the anger, at a conscious or a sub-conscious
level: 'Please, God, let me/him get better and I'll do this,
and that, and the other, for you ...'

The anger, and the pleas, are not answered. The natural
reaction is depression. This can hit you just when you
thought you were starting to get over it all, just when your
energy seems to be all spent already. Some people never get
out of this depression – patients, especially. They are alive
and they function, but they are not really living. Nothing is
worthwhile. If something like this stroke can happen, how
can there be any meaning to life? That's how they feel.

Depression is not a total disaster. It is, at least, a sign
that you are starting to absorb the reality of your situation,
even if you're over-reacting to it. You are processing information you will need for the rest of your life.

There's the potential for something better, after the
depression has been worked through. That's acceptance.
Heaven knows, you'd rather the stroke had not happened.
You're not completely crazy! But you have taken in the fact
that it *has* happened, and nothing you do will ever make it
un-happen. So you can at last start diverting your emotional
energy into making something out of life the way it is now,
and stop grieving all the time for life the way it was before.
You will have come to the end of a long, hard journey.

This is a general account of the grieving process – not a
recipe. It may be a bit different in your particular case. You
may skip a stage, or ricochet from one to another, or go backwards. Nobody can prescribe how long it all takes, either.
Some people get through it all quite quickly. Some take years.
Some stages take longer to work through than others.

Encouragement

Life is not a bowl of cherries, and things don't always progress without effort – quite a lot of effort. Both patient and carer need encouragement.

Encouragement is the art of focusing on assets and strengths – not liabilities. Discouragement is based on the belief that you are not adequate to deal with challenges. If you see yourself, or somebody else, as 'unable', what you usually get is inability. We tend to move in line with our expectations.

If you make a habit of focusing on the bad news, or mentally running yourself down, the effect is discouragement. So, every time you notice yourself doing it – just stop! If you catch yourself focusing on the nasty things your partner does, rather than the nice ones – again, stop!

It can take a long time to get out of the habit of focusing on the bad side. You'll catch yourself doing it again and again. But in time you'll learn to catch yourself *before* you focus on the bad, and re-focus on something more positive. It may seem silly, but it really will have an effect on how you feel – and act.

Learn, also, to separate the behaviour from the person. The fact that you have failed to do something to your complete satisfaction, or got it wrong, does not mean you are a bad person. You are an OK person who has got something wrong. Analyse the problem – not the person.

Carers need to make sure of encouragement, just as much as patients. The carer cannot instil confidence and faith in the patient if she does not have it herself. You cannot give something that you yourself do not have.

Personality changes?

'He's just not the same person he was before the stroke,' say some carers. And this can be the most upsetting thing of all. Sometimes it's hard to sort out physical causes from psychological causes.

For instance, personality traits which once were well controlled may now take the upper hand, either because of subtle damage within the brain or because of sheer stress. A man who didn't suffer fools gladly, and popped out for a smoke when he needed to cool down, now becomes a stick-banging tyrant. A quiet, rather passive woman becomes apathetic and drowned in self-pity.

Few adults like being told what to do, so many patients become stubborn and uncooperative. Others seem determined to retreat into themselves. They no longer consider other people's feelings; they hate themselves and the world.

Floods of tears and outbursts of temper are, of course, very common indeed. Rapid mood swings are partly caused by brain damage and partly by a normal human reaction to unbearable frustration and isolation.

The stroke patient has been likened to a combat veteran. He has been through terror; he has faced death; he is trapped in a situation which is not of his making. But, unlike the soldier, he has not been through all this with comrades at his side. He is completely alone. Some men came back from Vietnam and were never able to fit into their old life. It can happen to stroke patients, too.

If the carer finds in time that she cannot live with this new person, she has a right to be heard, and supported. A new personality in a familiar body means making a completely new relationship. Don't underestimate the upheaval this causes – it will be distressing and confusing. He has changed and you have stayed the same: how are you going to handle this unexpected situation? Going on with it, no matter what, is not the only option.

Some tips on feelings

- Don't feel bad about expressing your 'bad' feelings. Trying to suppress them increases their power, and it will show up in more destructive ways.
- But do keep the balance. The right to express bad feelings does not belong to one partner alone. One-sided complaining isn't fair, and doesn't work.
- Once you understand your bad feelings, you'll be able to see them coming the next time, learn the reason and get the support you need to cope with them.
- Remember to share the good feelings, too. You still love each other. You can share good times. You have good memories. You can celebrate progress towards recovery. Even a small improvement is worth celebrating.
- Don't think that any feeling you have is 'abnormal'. Almost certainly, it isn't. If you could talk frankly to someone who shares your situation, or if you could consult a psychologist, they'd be able to reassure you. Loneliness makes any feeling worse. So …
- Do talk to somebody about your feelings. Talk to each other, if you possibly can. Talk to an outsider, alone or together. Outsiders can bring a fresh point of view, or even see a funny side.
- It's no good just hoping things will get better if you're in a bad patch. They may not, unless you do something.
- Find your own, individualized coping strategies. What makes somebody else feel better won't necessarily work on you.

Tips for the carer

- Don't feel bad about expressing your own needs. The more clearly you can identify them, the better you can work out ways to fulfil them. The more fulfilled you are as a person, the better you will be as a carer.
- Don't be too idealistic about yourself. You're a human being, not a plaster saint.
- Don't resolve to be an absolute tower of strength, capable of coping with anything. Nobody is.
- Don't try to gloss over your feelings – least of all the 'bad' ones you think you shouldn't be having at all. Even Florence Nightingale got fed up sometimes.
- Don't be too shy to ask for help. As a carer, you have an important and very demanding job which makes you a very valuable person. The care you are giving would cost thousands if it were being done by a professional. You are entitled to support.
- Aim to get the patient doing more and more for himself. It's good for him, as well as you.
- Use the exercises in this book to help you identify exactly what help you need. Only then can you set about getting it.
- Look after your own needs – for fun, for peace and quiet, for company, for a life of your own. It will make you a better carer.

Anger and tears

Here are two feelings which interact like clockwork. You get angry; I burst into tears. You start crying over something silly; my patience snaps. Or, of course, the reflection can be direct: anger brings on anger; tears lead to tears. In fact, the two emotions are two sides of the same coin – frustration.

It's easy to see why the patient gets frustrated. He's suddenly become more helpless than he's ever been since babyhood – yet he still has all the intelligence and awareness that he's acquired as an adult. It's desperately lonely. It's very humiliating. And it all came out of nowhere, with no chance to prepare for it. Everything has gone out of control. Even his own body.

The carer reflects the same feeling of frustration. Her own life has been completely disrupted. The person she knew has suddenly turned into someone who depends on her almost as much as a baby. Her horizons have suddenly narrowed. Her life doesn't feel like her own any more. The patient has disappeared into a world of his own, which she can barely imagine. She feels so sorry for him. She feels helpless in the face of this catastrophe. It's confusing and painful – but the onus is on her to make it all right. She didn't choose this responsibility, any more than the patient chose to have a stroke. For her, too, everything is out of control.

The tears and anger come to the fore when the patient tries to do things. Of course he's frustrated when his body won't obey him even in the simplest things. He's wrestling with a useless piece of equipment which won't do the job any more. But he can't throw it down and do something else.

It's less appreciated that failure in small tasks is frustrating for the carer, too. She has to help and supervise him in doing things that both of them used to do without a second's thought. She's forced to drop down to his maddening, snail-like pace. She has to give the same guidance, and correct the same mistakes, over and over again. And she, at least, does have the physical power to go and do something else. She's only kept there by her own goodwill and self-discipline. She's quite likely to dissolve into anger and tears herself.

Coping strategies

- Don't take anger and tears personally. Even when they seem to be aimed at you, they probably aren't.
- Don't try to pretend that everything is fine, and nothing has changed. You both know that isn't true.
- Talk about the things that worry you. (Even if the patient can't talk to you, assume he can understand at least something of what you say. Don't block him out.)
- Be very clear in what you say to the patient. He has a lot of time to brood and get things out of proportion.
- Talk about your feelings. If you can both acknowledge them, they have less power over you. Anger and tears, in your circumstances, are a sign that you're both sane! They are very useful safety valves.
- Don't spend all your time delving into your psyche, though. If he bursts into tears because he's dropped his tea-cup, it's a lot more helpful to work out a way to stop him dropping it the next time. If he's too painfully frustrated by a task he's trying to master, see if it can be broken down into smaller, easier steps.
- Make a big fuss about successes. Neither of you is too old for a bit of child-like enthusiasm.

Follow your own feelings, at least sometimes. If both of you feel angry at once, have a good normal row. If you both feel like crying, cry together. It may be the best episode of communication you've managed all day.

- Devise outlets. The carer can leave the room and have a good howl, or thump cushions, or kick the wall, or just be alone. The patient should have the freedom and the privacy to do the same kind of things.
- If there has been a row, say sorry and make up afterwards. Normal people have rows and make up. You are still normal people.
- Realize that forgiving and forgetting are not the same thing. You'll probably be able to forgive, once you've been able to calm down and put yourself in the other person's shoes. Forgetting is too much to expect. Just forgive, and move on.
- Some things are pretty unforgivable. The carer might, for instance, do something that humiliates the patient in front of other people. The patient might be deliberately destructive (as far as you can tell). Tell the other person if he or she has gone too far. You both need to set some limits and establish some ground rules. Do so, and be consistent about them. You both need that kind of security.
- When you talk about feelings, talk about 'I' rather than 'you'. This means that the other person won't feel attacked – and won't need to become defensive. There's a lot of difference between 'I feel miserable' and 'You make me feel miserable'.
- Put five minutes aside at the end of your day to go over what happened together. Airing hurt and annoyance in time will stop them getting out of proportion.

Guilt and resentment

This unpleasant and powerful pair have their roots in the same frustrations which create anger and tears. Plus pity (and self-pity), plus the love between patient and carer.

Before going into the details, one thing has to be sorted out. When somebody has a stroke, it's common for the people around him to feel guilty about it. They think they must have brought it on – especially if there was a big upset or row shortly before the stroke happened. This guilt is misplaced. Strokes don't happen like that. In fact, about a fifth of strokes take place when the patient is peacefully asleep ...

Other feelings of guilt are harder to dismiss. Feelings of sin and guilt are built into our culture. They have their uses, in spurring us into action, but they can also be very destructive.

Women are particularly prone to guilt. They are brought up to look after everyone's needs but their own, to take the blame for a lot of things that go wrong and to feel it's their job to make things go better. If you have taken on the role of carer, you need to be very aware of the kind of pressure which may have led you to take on the job. People think it is 'natural' for a wife to care for her husband, and nobody expects her to do anything else – while a carer husband tends to be viewed with wonder and admiration. It's natural, where a spouse can't do the job, for the family eyes to fall on the nearest devoted daughter or kindly niece – especially if she isn't married ... Everyone concerned can be quite unconscious of the powerful assumptions which limit their thinking, and of the heavy pressures being exerted on a possibly reluctant volunteer.

Guilt can carry you *into* the role of carer, but it is not necessarily enough to carry you *through* it. Women, in particular, may have to think long and hard about their real motives for caring. It is not easy to do, and you may need help. Men, of course, are not immune to guilt either, and may have equally painful thinking to do.

Even where the caring role has been taken on willingly, and is fuelled by love, guilt is going to show up everywhere in the relationship between patient and carer. Many of these guilt feelings aren't rational at all, and the people who feel them know it. But they are nonetheless powerful, for all that. And all mixed up with guilt is the equally strong feeling of resentment.

The patient feels guilt for having had the stroke. Look what a burden he has become! Look at the havoc he has caused to the life of the carer! Look at the worry and expense he is causing! He is responsible for so much unhappiness and so much loss. He can no longer provide the things he used to provide – money, support, enjoyment, parenting for his children. He has created wide ripples of deprivation. His carer is being forced to neglect her own family; if the carer is his wife, he is depriving his own children and grandchildren.

At the same time, he is the victim of equally strong feelings of resentment. His family and carer have lost a lot, but he has lost a lot more. He can't help resenting their continued good health. What have they done to deserve their comparative good fortune? He can feel so sorry for himself that he resents any attempt by the carer to care for her own needs, or to get time off from caring for him. How dare she abandon him!

You can see how the vicious circle starts. Both the guilt and the resentment are irrational, and the patient knows it. His feelings of resentment give way to guilt that he is harbouring such feelings. In turn, the guilt becomes so unbearable that he cuts it off with its natural antidote – resentment ...

The same kind of circle is going around in the carer's mind. Her feelings are an exact mirror image of the patient's. She knows as well as he does what she has lost. She knows all about the havoc, the worry, the bills, and the burdens. But, of course, where the patient feels guilty, the carer feels resentment.

And just in the same way as it does in the patient's mind, in the carer's mind the resentment turns into guilt. How could she blame the poor patient for the effect his stroke has had on her? How could she be so selfish? How could she even think of her own needs, when he has been struck down and she still has her health and strength? Surely she should love him so much that she doesn't mind the sacrifices! Surely, whatever she is doing, she should do more! And when all this guilt becomes too much to bear, she snaps back into resentment.

Both patient and carer are reacting to the same facts, the same day-to-day worries. Each personal vicious circle draws power from the other.

Both guilt and resentment go deep and have a lot of power. They can't be reasoned away easily, because you already know they aren't reasonable. So put them in their place. They are very understandable, very natural, very common reactions to a painful situation. Learn to detect them. Spot them when they cause arguments. Then you can make a start on defusing them. Talk about them. They may be far too embarrassing and painful to broach with each other at first, so if you can't – don't let that cause further guilt or resentment! Talk to a sympathetic outsider, without your partner. Don't expect miraculous solutions to appear. You just need to talk and talk until the feelings lose some of their power. Other patients, and other carers, are certain to understand these feelings and to share them. That will make it a lot easier for you, and give you some resources to help you in approaching your partner.

Guilt and resentment take a lot of coming to terms with. As you explore them, you may find that in your case, their origins go deeper than the stroke itself. Their power may come from older guilts and resentments, woven into your relationship long ago. If your relationship wasn't perfect before, a stroke isn't likely to improve it. Try to get expert help if old problems are leading to new problems now.

Your first priority will be to tackle the practical problems caused by the guilt-resentment cycle. The most important one of these is likely to be the carer's difficulty in dividing her attention between the patient, other people who depend on her – and herself. Solving this problem can't be left to chance.

In the meantime, comfort yourself with two thoughts. First, only nice people feel guilty – selfish and uncaring people don't suffer from guilt. Second, feelings of guilt have no connection with the actual degree of guilt. A mass murderer may feel no guilt at all, while most of us can feel a crippling guilt when we have done nothing to earn such a feeling at all.

How to talk

It isn't easy to talk about feelings. Even in our closest relationships, many of us lost the habit years ago. The easiest way to get started is to set aside five minutes, for each of you, at the end of the day, to do a review of the day and get feelings out. Make it part of your routine. The old advice is still valid: don't go to sleep on a quarrel.

In order for this idea to work, you have to agree it first. It can be set up as part of the day's structure: 'Why don't we take some time each day just to look back and say how we feel about what went on? Each of us can have five whole minutes. Can we agree on that?' (You'll be amazed, by the way, at how much can be said in five minutes!) This will stop things from festering. If, however, there's something you really don't want to talk about, you need to take conscious responsibility for not doing that.

One very useful thing a carer can try is to 'model' the kind of thing you want. If a carer starts doing something, probably the patient will follow suit – in time. One thing a carer can model is saying: 'I feel ...', and making a point of saying 'I feel' rather than 'I think'. This gives the patient permission to feel, and permission to say how she feels.

Another thing the carer can model is talking about positive things. If it's been a day of gloom and despair, find something positive to mention before you go to bed. If only one thing went right today, mention it. Even one good thing is better than nothing. It wasn't a great day, but at least she managed to hold a cup with more tea in it than yesterday ... Little things count, and there's probably some little thing that happened during the day which needs to be focused on.

Important in all of this is your motivation. You have to want to make things better. The difficulty is that, for a while, the carer might find herself alone in being positive. The patient is so involved in her own experience, and her own disability, that she is not ready or willing to look at anything positive. You have to go on despite it.

A final technique, which might be useful, takes courage. This is 'grasping the nettle'. If you think that something is going on, if you think the patient is upset or depressed or annoyed or fed up, sit down, make a gesture of affection (like squeezing her hand), and say something like: 'I notice you're being quiet ... I notice you're not looking at me ... and I wonder if something's wrong. I wonder if I've done something wrong, and I wonder if you're feeling unhappy ... '

The difficult thing is that you might get a 'yes', of course. Yes, I feel miserable. Yes, there's no hope. But it's worthwhile taking the risk and bringing it out into the open. It's better that feelings are talked about than sat on. Take a risk and make a guess about what might be going on.

Choose your moment. Not when either of you is tired, or when there are other people around, or when the big game is about to come up on TV. If you have had an argument, or one of you has had a fit of temper, wait for it to die down. Then go in with your: 'Is there something that we need to talk about?' Don't doom your attempt to failure by coming in too soon after the fight, or picking a moment when there's no time to talk properly. Set time aside for it.

Good times

This section has dealt with unpleasant, uncomfortable emotions – for the very good reason that people seldom seek help in 'coping' with pleasant feelings. Just don't get the idea that caring is all doom and gloom. It is, more often than not, a very rewarding experience which deepens the relationship between carer and cared-for.

You learn a lot about each other, and about life. You can see – in yourself and in the other person – courage and strength and love of a depth you would never have known was possible if life had continued in the way you had planned. Your horizons are expanded, not diminished.

You learn to cherish and savour the good times together. You appreciate them a hundred times more, because they have been created by you, not handed over on a plate.

Crisis and change are the beginning of something new – if we allow them to be. Crisis and change are destructive only when we resist them, hold on to old ways and try to continue just as we did before, no matter what. Seen properly, dealt with honestly, they give you a chance to break old rules, find new powers and create something very special.

Workbook 3

The workbook has two quizzes:

ARE YOU OVER-STRESSED?
and
WHAT'S THE PROBLEM?
They are easy to do, although they may arouse painful thoughts. They will identify what's really bothering you. The quizzes are for both patient and carer to use. Comparing notes will be very interesting ...

The next part is harder work. It is a method for solving the problems you have identified, so it's obviously worth trying. It may give you some good ideas. It is called:

ACTION PLANNING
The final part of the workbook is a choice of:

MIND GAMES
Unless you are terribly serious all the time, at least one of these games will be easy to play – and quite helpful and informative. Pick whichever one you fancy. As usual, you start with the easiest thing. Do them all if you like.

If you *are* being terribly serious all the time, try to give it a break. The games might spark something off. A sense of humour is one of the nicest ways of coping with a stroke, and if you can help give one back to the patient you are doing a lot for him. You can't give a sense of humour if you haven't got one yourself. You might even enjoy the occasional laugh.

This exercise can be used by both patient and carer. Best of all, you can both do it and compare notes.

ARE YOU OVER-STRESSED?

This exercise helps you keep tabs on your stress level, and to be aware when it's getting too high for comfort. The sooner you realize what's happening, the sooner you can do something about it.

Don't just do this exercise once and then forget about it. Do it regularly. Things change. Your ability to cope varies.

Everyone reacts to over-stress in different ways. By doing this exercise regularly, you'll learn to get in touch with your own individual stress signs. The signs listed all affect us to some degree. You are looking for things which affect you *too much*. If you find it difficult, give each sign a score out of 10. A score over 7 is too much!

Physical stress signs
- Aches and pains: head-ache, neck and shoulder tension, back pain, other pains
- Frequent minor illness: coughs and colds, indigestion, diarrhoea, others
- Fatigue
- Disturbed sleep
- Weight loss or weight gain
- Overeating or undereating
- Chemical dependence: tobacco, alcohol, other drugs.

Psychological stress signs
- Boredom
- Sexual problems
- Impulsive acts
- Crying
- Depression
- Irritability
- Anger
- Others (look for any departure from the behaviour you think of as typically 'you').

Social stress signs
- Rows with the patient/carer
- Rows with friends or relatives
- Rows with professionals
- Blaming other people for everything
- Acts of unkindness
- Avoiding the patient or carer as much as you can
- Avoiding other people
- Others.

WHAT'S THE PROBLEM?

This exercise is for patients. If the patient has no language, the carer may have ways to question him, or observe him, and do it on his behalf as best she can.

This book can't possibly list all the things that could be over-stressing you. But *you* know what they are, deep down inside. Now you need to bring them to the surface and really pin them down.

This might be very difficult. You might not want to admit some of the things you are feeling — even to yourself. This checklist gives you some starter ideas. Be assured that they have been put on the list because they are very common. There is nothing abnormal about you if you feel the same way.

- The carer is not the same person he/she used to be.
- The carer doesn't understand your problems.
- The carer understands your problems, but has no sympathy.
- The carer ignores your needs.
- The carer makes you work too hard.
- The carer has all the power.
- The carer is making a mess of jobs that you used to do.
- The carer treats you like a baby or an idiot.
- The carer *enjoys* treating you like a baby or an idiot.
- You hate having certain things done to you: being cleaned up, washed, fed, helped to the lavatory, others.
- The carer doesn't love you any more.
- The carer secretly wants to abandon you.
- The carer wishes you were dead.
- You can't communicate with anyone.
- People talk in front of you as if you can't understand – and you don't like the things they say.
- You get angry all the time because of the things you can't do.
- You cry all the time because of all the things you can't do.
- You feel frustrated, especially by …?
- You hate being prey to emotions and unable to control them.
- Your stroke has ruined everything for your carer and/or family.
- You are worried sick about money.
- You miss the life you had before the stroke.
- You feel bitter about the plans and dreams for the future which can never come true.

- You feel cut off from the real world.
- You feel trapped.
- You are not the same person you used to be.
- You are not getting better as much, or as fast, as you had hoped.
- You're afraid of things that never used to bother you.
- You feel guilty that the carer can't attend to her own family as she should.
- You feel guilty that you are unable to be a parent to your children any more.
- You feel that friends and family are not giving enough support.
- You feel that professionals are not giving enough support.
- You feel that the stroke is your own fault.
- You have conflicting feelings which confuse you: love and hate for the carer, resentment and gratitude, hope and despair, others.
- You hate being a burden.
- You're afraid you will go mad.
- You're tired, tired, tired.
- You feel unattractive and unlovable.
- You don't like your body.
- You feel things will never get any better.
- You wish you were dead.
- Other worries about people's behaviour.
- Other practical problems.
- Other feelings within yourself.

WHAT'S THE PROBLEM?
This exercise is for carers.

This book can't possibly list all the things that could be over-stressing you. But *you* know what they are, deep down inside. Now you need to bring them to the surface and really pin them down.

This might be very difficult. You might not want to admit some of the things you are feeling – even to yourself. This checklist gives you some starter ideas. Be assured that they have been put on the list because they are very common. There is nothing abnormal about you if you feel the same way.

- The patient is not the same person he/she used to be.
- The patient makes demands on you all the time.
- The patient doesn't seem to care how you feel at all.
- The patient doesn't like being cared for by anyone but you. You can't get a break.
- The patient has habits which irritate you: dribbling, talking nonsense, constant crying, others.
- You can't help feeling revolted by some of the things you have to do: humouring the patient, washing intimate parts, feeding him, cleaning up after incontinence, helping him in the lavatory, others.
- The patient gets angry with you.
- The patient gets upset when he tries to do things and fails.
- You can't have a conversation with the patient.
- The patient won't co-operate with important things that must be done to get him better.
- The patient isn't getting better as much, or as fast, as you'd hoped.
- You feel desperately sorry for the patient.
- You feel you're not doing enough for the patient.
- You feel you're doing too much for the patient.
- You don't love the patient enough (or at all!).
- You miss the life you had before the stroke.
- You're worried sick about money.
- You feel cut off from the real world.

- You feel trapped.
- You feel you can't possibly cope with all the responsibilities you have.
- You feel that friends and family have been only too happy to put the whole burden on to you.
- You feel jealous of people who seem happier and more free than you.
- You feel that professionals are not giving you enough support.
- You have conflicting feelings which confuse you: love and hate for the patient, resentment and guilt at feeling resentful, anger and pity, others.
- You're afraid you will go mad.
- You're afraid you'll never have a life of your own again.
- You're tired, tired, tired.
- You feel things will never get any better.
- You wish the patient was dead.
- You wish you were dead.
- Other worries about the patient's behaviour.
- Other practical problems.
- Other feelings within yourself.

ACTION
This exercise is for both patient and carer to do, either separately or together,

Filling in the **What's the problem?** checklist is already action. Do it regularly, to keep tabs on your situation and your emotional health. Listing the current problems means you are aware of them. You may have found the exercise upsetting.

Step 1 Don't bury that pain. Have a good cry, a good scream or whatever you can do to release some of it. You need to do this for your own sake and each other's sake. And don't tell yourself: 'I've had my cry/screaming session now. That's enough.' Go along with those emotions whenever they come up, and whenever you get the chance. This will lessen their power to overwhelm you.

Step 2 Now – what next? You've identified some problems. That's the first step towards solving them. Next step is to put them in some kind of order.

- Some problems have a practical solution, if you think about it. For instance, there may be ways to make unpleasant tasks easier, or to get the patient to take them over. You need know-how.
- Some problems can be eased by information. Why does the patient behave as he does? Are there any tips for coping?
- Some problems are to do with your whole relationship – the one you had before the stroke, and the one you've got now. How can you explore these depths?
- Some problems tell you something about your own needs as a person. Can you be more precise about what those needs are, and what is stopping them from being fulfilled?

Rule of Thumb: look at each problem in turn, and see if it can be re-framed as a practical problem which could be solved with specific information and advice. This kind of help is often the easiest to ask for and to get.

Step 3 Identify your priorities. You probably have quite a list of problems by now. Most people do. You can't work on all of them at once. Put a mark against the problems which worry you most:

- Never mind what you think you *ought* to worry about most. Something seemingly quite silly might be your personal last straw. If someone tells you a problem or a feeling is silly, that person is a lot sillier than you are.
- Don't fool yourself. You may want to put a certain problem at the bottom of the list because the thought of tackling it is more than you can face, or it seems too hopeless to have a solution. If you can face up to it, you may be pleasantly surprised by the result.

Step 4 Identify who might help. Look through the resources section to identify professionals, organizations and ordinary people who might help.

- Be flexible. For instance, the most helpful professional might not be the most obvious one, but the one who gets on best with you.
- Be bold. People won't break into little pieces if you approach them for help and advice. They might even be flattered. They might even come up with the help you need!
- Make a start. You may be faced with a problem and not have a clue who is the best person to help. So ask someone else to suggest who *can* help.

Step 5 Seek out the help you need.

- Make a note of what the problem is, in case your mind goes blank at the crucial time and you miss out some significant detail. You may even need to gather up proof. If your dear old white-haired mother sometimes behaves with unbelievable violence, for instance, make a tape recording. You can be sure she won't perform to order;

you *can't* be sure that potential helpers won't dismiss your complaint as exaggerated.

- Make a note of any suggested solution. It's very easy to forget some of the details, especially if you are under stress. You need to know exactly what to do.
- Check that the suggested solution is practical. It's sometimes tempting to say 'thank you' and back out although you are not satisfied – especially if the problem you have brought up embarrasses you. Is the solution something you are able to carry out? If you are advised to buy something, can you afford it?

Step 6 Carry out the suggested solution.
This seems a silly thing to say, but sometimes it's easier to find the energy to moan about something than it is to do something positive about it.

Step 7 See if it worked.
Again, this seems a silly thing to say. But it's difficult to keep track of everything that's going on, and sometimes people forget to follow through. Check against your original list.

Step 8 If it didn't work, start again.
Don't despair. If the problem is still bothering you, you shouldn't just decide you must live with it somehow. Another solution may be possible.

Step 9 If it did work, congratulate yourself! Then move on to another problem.

SEVEN MIND GAMES
Sometimes you need a fresh point of view. Sometimes you need extra insight into an everyday situation. Sometimes

you need to release the power of your imagination. These ideas may seem crazy, but they work – for both patient and carer. They certainly make a change from being serious all the time ...

- Write a job description for your role as patient or carer. What are the duties? The pay-offs? The qualities required to hold down the job? What insights does this give you?
- Write a biography of yourself or the patient/carer. What kind of person is this? What are his/her interests? How has he/she coped with crises in the past? What insights does this give you?
- Write a letter to yourself, the patient/carer, your former self, the patient/carer as s/he used to be, or anyone else you wish you could sort things out with. Be 100 per cent honest. You probably won't want to post it, but you'll feel better, and may learn something useful.
- Listen to the 'inner voices' you hear, telling you how you feel or what you 'ought' to feel or do. Is it a voice, a feeling, a picture, or ...? Is it inside you, or coming from outside? Does it remind you of a person or a situation? What does this tell you?
- Re-work those inner messages, as if you were a media producer. Make dark pictures brighter, make threatening figures do something ridiculous, make positive voices louder, negative voices soft, squeaky ... whatever you find that makes you feel better.
- Act 'as if'. Retreat into pretending you're a nurse, a therapist, a war hero (etc.) when there are unpleasant tasks to be done. Try play-acting some of the things you think you'd like to be, or ought to be – Housewife, Superstar, the brave patient, the assertive person who can deal with put-downs, the saint. Play-acting is a way

of trying new attitudes without making grim resolutions, experimenting with hidden powers, making relationships more bearable – or just having fun.

- See what you learn by imagining the other person as an animal (cuddly bear? big bad wolf? pig?), or film star (Stan Laurel? Oliver Hardy? Greta Garbo?), or fictional character (Scrooge? Peter Pan? Captain Ahab?), or real person (St Sebastian? Florence Nightingale? Guy Fawkes?) and so on. Picture yourself in the same ways.

5

MOVEMENT

This section aims to guide you through all the stages from sitting in a chair to getting into a car. While every stroke patient will want and need to sit in a chair, not everyone will want to do all the work involved in learning all the skills in this section. Some are very old; some remain very disabled.

Very elderly patients may simply choose not to take things much further, and not take on the effort of learning to walk again. Other patients will remain too badly disabled to walk, whether they want to or not. Many patients will benefit by building up an interesting wheelchair life before moving on to walking. It all depends on the individual. Most things in stroke care do!

Patient and carer need to look at the future lifestyle they want and can manage. It is probably some time now since the stroke happened, and both of you are out of the first, numbing shock which fell on you in the first days or weeks. It is time to reassess.

You certainly need professional help in doing this, and the professional in question is the physiotherapist. You need some kind of realistic basis for your own assessment of what you want, what you are prepared to do to get it. Many patients, of course, make a complete recovery without much trouble. Others will have to work hard to make the same kind of progress.

Some patients will have to settle for less than complete recovery – much less, in some cases. Too much of the brain has been damaged. Unfortunately, there are patients who simply cannot believe this. It is better to be optimistic than pessimistic, and the casebooks are full of examples of people who astounded their doctors by their progress. But completely unrealistic expectations can cause a lot of pain and bitterness. Sometimes, of course, it is the carer and not the patient who has to be persuaded that miracles are unlikely to happen. Patients can be made very unhappy if they are nagged and pushed to achieve the impossible.

For other patients and carers, the problem is just the opposite. The patient gives up hope, when further progress is in fact well within his capabilities. His confidence and self-esteem have been shattered, and he is afraid to try. Full-blown depression is a natural reaction in someone who has had a stroke. Sometimes the damage to the brain is itself a cause of depression. Antidepressants may or may not help. Motivating such a patient is a nightmare for the carer, and no carer can be expected to cope with it alone.

Assessment by the physiotherapist is the first step towards getting to grips with these problems. How much progress is likely, given the patient's type of stroke and degree of handicap? If patient and carer disagree about their expectations, the physiotherapist is in the best position to help them sort it out.

The physiotherapist is the person who will design a programme of exercise to maximize recovery, and will teach the best way for each individual patient (and carer) to tackle tasks like standing and walking.

Traditionally, the patient's friends and family were given no role to play. But it is acknowledged more and more, today, that they can do a lot. The patient will need skilled teaching and therapy sessions. But constant practice is the real key to progress.

Patients get very tired, especially when they are trying to master a new skill, so they will have to get into the habit of short, frequent practice at home, with regular access to a physiotherapist who can check that mistakes are not creeping in, and suggest further activities as milestones are reached and passed.

The text that follows, then, is only a guide and not a set of absolute rules. Different physiotherapists have different opinions on some of the details. In order to keep up a consistent pattern of work, you should follow your own therapist's advice on these details.

Be safe
Helping a patient about involves a certain amount of supporting him. This puts a strain on the carer's body very similar to the strain of lifting. So before you go any further, turn back to Section 3, **Early days,** and make sure the basic principles of safe lifting have become second nature. And ask the physiotherapist for some more tips.

CHAIR EXERCISES
You have now come a long way from the helpless patient lying in bed and the harassed carer doing everything for him. The next steps are complex and need to be supervised by a physiotherapist.

UPPER HALF

You will want to go on developing power and balance
above the waist. A few more exercises will help. For the
first two, you need a table. A mirror will also help.

1 Bending forward

Remove any pillows from the table. Get the patient to
interlace his fingers, with help if necessary. Place feet well
back under the chair. Now the patient should slide his
hands forward across the table, bending forward. The
further the better. Now reverse the process until he is
sitting upright again. Then get him to raise his arms above
his head. This is hard work, as the weak arm is heavy.

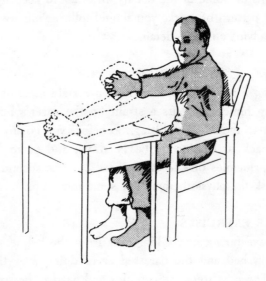

2 Arm swings

Interlace the fingers and swing both arms from side to
side. Start with arms on the table, then gradually raise
them – first, just clear of the table, and then higher and

higher until the patient can do them sitting upright. All this is good progress. Patient and carer must make sure they get a pat on the back as higher and higher swings are achieved. But don't go too high – anything above shoulder level can be damaging.

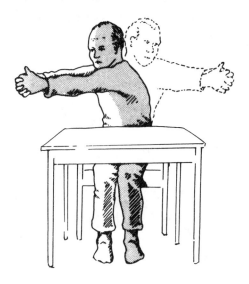

3 Bending down

Now remove the table from in front of the patient. Fingers interlaced once again, he should lean forward and try to reach down to his feet. Balance is important, and he should not lean over to one side or the other. It is a good idea to watch the hands – but not to let the head drop right forward on to the chest. As he improves, he can put his hands on the outside of his legs and slide them down towards his ankles. Again, it is easy to note progress, as hands reach lower and lower down the legs. And each bit of progress is cause for congratulation.

GETTING TO THE CHAIR INDEPENDENTLY

Look back to **Do-it-yourself sitting** and **Moving from bed to chair** in Section 3 (page 70). The same basic method is used when the patient gets himself into the chair without help – with the same points to watch for. The difference this time is that the patient leans, not on the carer, but on his own hand (the strong one), which is placed flat on the bed close to his side.

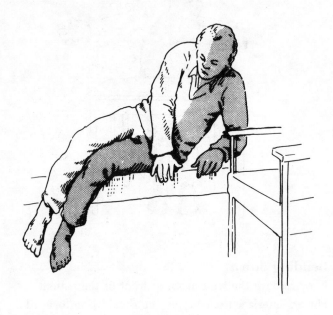

- The most important thing is to lean forward all the time, until the patient is firmly seated. He should not even look up until then!
- The first few times, both patient and carer will probably feel nervous. The carer should be close at hand with the hand nearest the bed at his waist, and the other hand on his shoulder, making sure he leans forward.

- If things go wrong, turn to **What if he falls?** on page 126!
- At first, the non-affected leg will take his weight as he pivots round. Make sure this habit wears off as the affected side of the body gets stronger. It must learn to play its full part again.

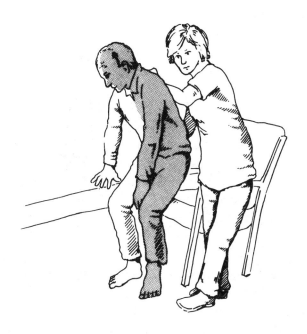

STANDING UP

Standing up is well within the power of just about every stroke patient. It is an important skill to acquire, for the carer's sake. Without it, all kinds of normal daily activities become difficult – moving from bed to chair (or commode, or lavatory), dressing, washing.

It is also a vital stage in rehabilitating the patient back to normal movement. After all, it is all about balance and using both halves of the body equally.

Finally, it's a great way to relieve pressure on the body which could still be in danger of causing pressure sores.

If you have done all the chair exercises you are well placed to start standing. To get out of a chair, you need to do three things:

- move to the edge of the seat
- place feet well back, under the chair
- lean forward

IDEAL STANDING METHOD
With luck, the carer will need to give no help at all. At most, she should stand in front of the patient to give him confidence, and place her hands on his shoulder blades to make sure he keeps leaning forward (it's almost impossible to get up without leaning forward, even if you have no handicap at all. Try it and see!)

The patient's job is to:

- sit with weight evenly balanced over the two halves of the body
- have knees bent, with feet flat on the floor
- put the weak foot a little behind the unaffected foot, to make sure that weight will be taken by the weak leg
- lean well forward from the hips
- clasp hands and stretch the arms out in front
- lift hips off the floor, still leaning forward and ...
- stand
- now celebrate this important achievement!

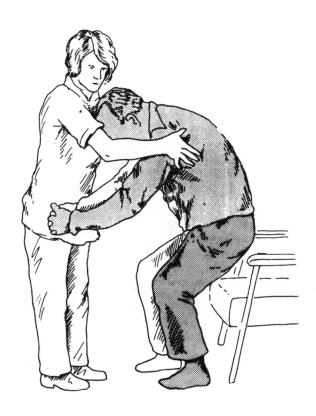

ALTERNATIVE METHOD

Some patients will find they need to use an easier method. This involves using the good arm to push up on the chair. It is not ideal, because it is always best to use the affected (weak) side as much as possible, to keep the body balanced and encourage maximum recovery. But standing up is important, and should start as soon as possible using what-ever method does the trick.

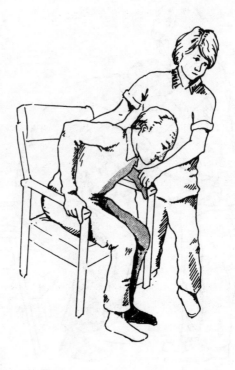

So don't get into the habit of using this method. Try the 'ideal method' from time to time, to see if the patient is ready for it. Patients must do as much as possible, in all things, and carers should do as little as possible.

The patient's job is to:

• sit as before, but with the good hand on the arm of the chair

- place his weak foot a little behind the unaffected one, as before
- lean well forward
- push down with the hand and stand up.

The carer's job is to:

- stand at the patient's weak side
- hold his affected hand on the chair arm. This helps the patient keep a more even balance and not slump over
- use the other hand to help the patient lean forward
- **don't** put your hand under the patient's armpit on the weak side. The shoulder is still vulnerable.

Sitting

IDEAL METHOD
This is a simple reversal of the standing up method. Make sure, of course, that the chair is right behind the patient – he should be able to check this for himself by feeling it against the back of his legs.

The patient's job is to:

- place the weak foot slightly behind the other, so the affected leg takes some weight
- clasp his hands and stretch his arms out in front
- lean well forward, with head forward
- lower on to the chair.

If necessary, the carer can place her hands on his shoulder blades, as with standing up, to keep the patient leaning forward and guide his direction.

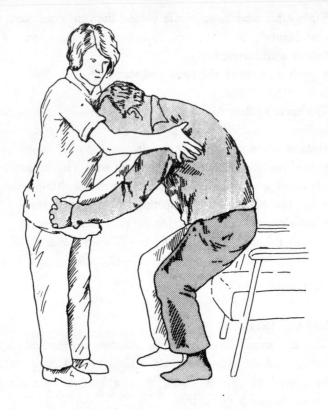

ALTERNATIVE SITTING METHOD

Again, this is a simple reversal of the alternative standing up method. Again, it is a method to be used only as long as it is necessary. Check regularly to see if the patient can now manage the ideal method.

The patient's job is to:

- stand close in front of the chair, as above
- hold the chair arm with the unaffected hand
- lean well forward
- lower onto the chair

If necessary, the carer stands at his weak side, holding his weak hand on the chair arm to make sure he doesn't slump over to the other side.

STANDING WELL
Good position and balance will always be important, no matter how much progress the patient makes. The patient may be afraid he will fall on his affected side, and so put all his weight on the good side. He needs to train himself to stand with:

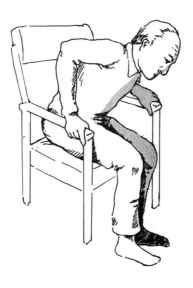

- head in line with the spine, not tilted
- shoulders level
- hips level
- feet level and flat on the floor.

The patient is also likely to have trouble with his weak leg. It may be floppy and give way at the knee or ankle. On the other hand it may 'lock' straight at the knee and refuse to bend as he tries to walk. The resulting strain on the knee causes damage.

STANDING PLUS ...

Standing is the ideal basis for practising things that will help the patient to balance on his legs, to use his weak side more and to use his unaffected side (both arm and leg) in a normal way – not using non-normal movements in an attempt to 'compensate' for the weak side. Remember, you are not aiming to move in a new way but to re-learn the old, balanced way. You *must* get expert advice from the physiotherapist on just what to do. Basically, it's about transferring his weight from side to side, and using his weak arm to the full.

WHAT IF HE FALLS?

A fall is not the end of the world, except in a very frail patient who should not be put at risk by trying to progress too fast. For most patients, a fall or two may well happen. Nobody should feel guilty about this. The only way to make absolutely sure of not falling is never to try to move at all. Normal life is full of risks, and life after a stroke is still normal life – or should be.

If you fall on to your back:

- stretch out (or, if necessary, lift) the weak arm away from the body
- bring the strong arm across the body
- bend the strong leg and lift it over the other one
- roll over onto the weak side.

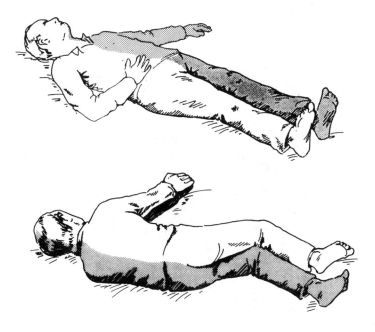

If you fall on your side, you are already halfway to getting up. From a side position:

- bend the sound leg
- put the sound arm on the floor
- push up until you are on all fours.

If you fall face downwards:

- bend the sound leg
- push down with the sound hand until you are on all fours.

GETTING UP FROM ALL FOURS

Now you need a chair. Someone should bring one and put it in front of you. Now:

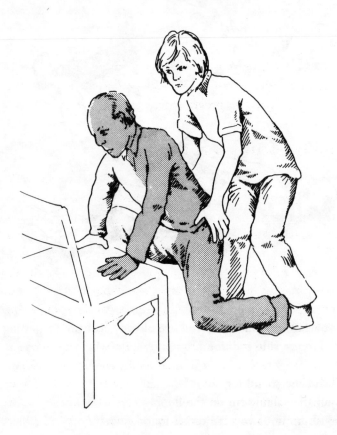

- put your hands on the seat
- bring the strong leg forward, bend the knee and put the foot flat on the floor
- lean forward and push up onto your feet
- pivot round, perhaps with help, and sit down.

If there's nobody to bring a chair, you may be able to rock your way on your buttocks to get to one, in the same way you learned to move on the bed. If you are near the stairs, you may be able to push yourself up to sit on the bottom step, then the next one, then the next one, until you are high enough to stand.

Falling is frightening; getting up is very tiring. Have a rest and do whatever is most likely to make you feel calm again. Please don't be put off. After a decent interval, get back to your exercise programme.

Standing with an aid

The ideal to aim for is to walk *without* a stick, using a well-balanced body. For old or frail patients (or old and frail helpers!), this may simply be too much to take on. Walking with a stick, or some other aid, has disadvantages: the good hand is occupied and can't do anything else. It may also encourage a limping walk. But you may find it's a choice between this kind of walking and no walking at all. Patient, carer and physiotherapist should discuss just how high you should aim.

By now, you and the physiotherapist will have made a decision on whether to go for unaided standing or walking, or whether to use an aid. This aid may be a stick. Or it may be a walking frame (preferably one with wheels, so it does not have to be lifted up to move forward). With either type of aid, its height is very important. Too low, and it will cause strain and imbalance. Its top should be level with the patient's wrist when her arm is bent at an angle of about 90° (a right angle).

STANDING WITH A FRAME
- The patient stands behind the frame, feet pointing forward.
- She puts both hands on the frame, making sure she puts weight on her weak arm and leg.
- The carer stands behind her, at her weak side.
- For extra help, the carer can put his arm across the patient's back and his hand on her unaffected hip.
- If the patient's knee is still unstable, the carer can steady it with his own.

STANDING WITH A STICK
- The patient stands with feet pointing forward.
- She holds the stick in her good hand.
- The carer stands at her weak side, one arm round her waist, the other across her back and resting on her sound hip.
- If the patient's weak knee is unstable, the carer can brace it with his own.
- Later, the carer can stand further away and give support by holding the patient's weak arm – elbow straight, hand flat.

NEXT STEPS
This book does not contain advice or pictures about getting the patient to walk. There is a good reason for this. Re-learning the ability to walk is quite a complex business.

It is the physiotherapist's job. It is not an area for

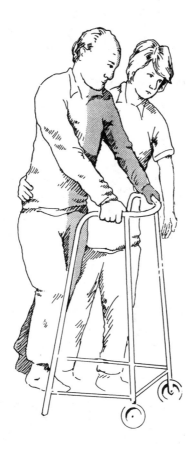

well-meaning amateurs to have a go. The physio won't be keen for the patient to try walking for himself (even with a carer's help) until he has had a lot of practice under her supervision.

Walking involves a lot of physical skills and capacities, which have to be broken down into small stages and mastered one by one. Also – as always! – no two stroke

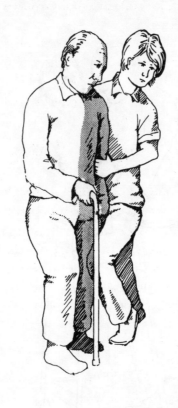

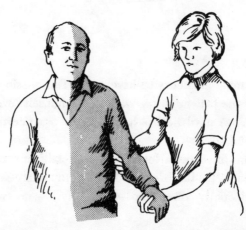

patients are alike. Each will have to overcome a slightly different set of problems.

Often, he will also have his own personal set of perception problems to deal with – not being aware that the weak side of his body exists at all, not being able to judge space or distance, and so on. These perception problems can be more disabling than the physical imbalances.

The physiotherapist should be doing a certain amount of work with the patient on his own – either in the hospital Physio department or at a day centre or similar. He or she will do various rhythmic and balancing movements with the patient in various positions – lying down, sitting, standing or even kneeling.

As always, the aim will be to get the body back in balance, and able to function in as normal a way as possible. At the right time – and not before – the physiotherapist will help the patient transfer his weight from leg to leg, to stand on one leg and swing the other back and forth in a walking motion, and so on until he is walking.

Your job, in the meantime, is to keep the patient as mobile as possible without accidentally causing any damage to him, or – every bit as important – to yourself.

Watch the physiotherapist work as often as you can, ask questions and be ready to help out when the time comes.

WHEELCHAIRS

Most stroke patients find themselves in a wheelchair at some stage. For many, it will be a transitional stage which allows them independence, and gives the carer a break, while the long haul to walking goes on. A trip to the garden or the shops is thus possible right from the start, and at home the patient may be able to move himself about using a hand-propelled or motorized model.

Beware temptation. A wheelchair can be so much easier than trying to get about under one's own steam. It is tempting to use it indoors quite a lot. For the patient who is likely to make a good recovery, this is a tragedy. He starts to go backwards; mobility reduces and deformities may be caused.

Beware something else – pressure sores. An advantage of having to move about on one's feet is that pressure is taken off the buttocks. Pressure sores can easily be caused by wheelchairs. Take advice on proper padding and cushions. The paralysed patient should also raise himself out of the seat at least every half hour, to restore blood flow in the pressure area.

Some stroke patients will never leave their wheelchairs. If the handicap remains severe, walking will never be possible. Many older patients take the view that they have worked hard all their lives and don't want any more of it, even if they are capable of walking. Many older carers will feel relieved by this decision! It should be discussed with a professional if possible, but it is a perfectly reasonable decision to take. Not all of us want to push forward the frontiers of human endeavour ...

A whole book could easily be devoted to wheelchairs. New models come out almost daily, including quite revolutionary designs. Some have to be pushed; some are self-propelled, which is much better for the patient and the carer. Some are motorized. Some can climb kerbs and hills and go on for miles. Some are like little cars. There are light, sporty models which fold up and can be carried in a car. There are indoor models which might even be small enough to get through doors.

Free wheelchairs are provided if you qualify for state aid. They are not, unfortunately, always the best available. But the best wheelchairs cost money. If you can lay hands on the money for a better model, it could be well worth it. If you are thinking of buying, get lots and lots of advice from an occupational therapist or disability adviser. Good manufacturers will probably let you have a model on trial. The wrong wheelchair is an expensive disaster.

CAR TRAVEL

Patient and carer both need to get outdoors. They both need to remember there is a world outside their own private one. Car trips are possible from quite an early stage. If you have no car, take up a car-owning friend's offer of help, or seek out a local church or voluntary group.

You'll need to think about where you are going. Access to public buildings is often appalling, and you will need to check this in advance. A drive in the country is an easier and very refreshing alternative until you have the right information at your fingertips. Public lavatories for disabled people are also thin on the ground, so unless you are sure take a urinal and a blanket for privacy, or resort to incontinence pads if you have no alternative.

If you have a choice of cars, a two-door car is usually easier to get into than a four-door model. In either case, the best seat is the front passenger seat. Move the seat as far back as possible and recline it slightly, to give maximum space for manoeuvre. The higher the seat, the better. A firm cushion might help if the seat seems rather low. Try it out before the patient tries it, to get an idea.

Have the car parked away from the kerb, so the patient can stand in the road, and open the car door fully. The patient turns his back on the car. He bends forwards and lowers himself as far back on to the seat as possible, with help if necessary. Remember the lifting rules if help is given

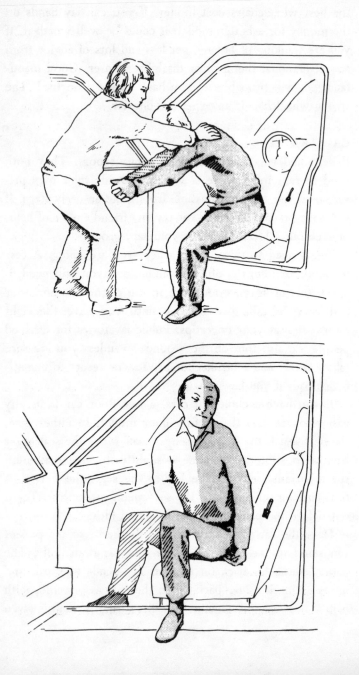

– back straight, knees bent, feet apart. Make sure the patient's head does not hit the door frame. Then the patient moves further on to the seat by rolling from hip to hip. The carer lifts one leg in, then the other. Even better, the patient does this himself. This is easier if he leans backwards. The patient turns to face the front, with help if necessary. Don't forget to lock the door and put on the seat belt. Many patients can do this for themselves. To get out of the car, carry out all the same steps in reverse. Remember the patient should lean well forward, to make the moves easier and avoid banging his head. If the patient needs help standing up, he should place his arms on the carer's shoulders.

Don't grip the patient at the armpit on the affected side. Put your arm around his shoulder, on the outside.

MOVING FROM WHEELCHAIR TO CAR

Longer expeditions are possible for early stroke patients who can take a wheelchair with them on a car trip. There are special wheelchairs and car fitments which allow the patient to transfer herself, and state aid may be available. But here is the method for getting from an ordinary wheelchair into an ordinary car.

Park the car far enough from the kerb to make room for the wheelchair. Open the car door, move the wheelchair footrest nearest the car out of the way, and place the wheelchair as close as possible to the car, facing the front. Use a blanket or piece of foam rubber to protect the car's paintwork. Lock the wheelchair brakes and adjust the footrests out of the way.

The patient leans forward, feet flat on the ground, and pushes with her arms to stand up. She turns her back on the car. Depending on which side is the weak one, she can steady herself on the arm of the wheelchair, the car's door

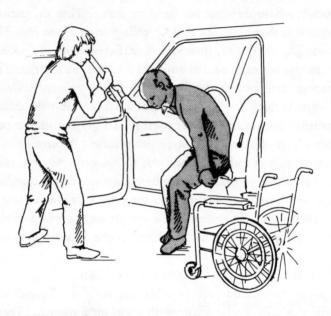

frame or window frame. Someone must hold the car door steady if it is being used in this way. The patient lowers herself on the car seat, as far back on it as possible. She must still lean forward and guard against banging her head on the door frame. She lifts her legs inside, one by one, or the carer does it for her.

To get back from the car into the wheelchair, use the same procedure in reverse. Check that the wheelchair's brakes are on. Getting out of the car, the patient is more likely to need support to stand up.

DRIVING
Some stroke patients are keen to drive again. Even if full power does not return to the weak side, there are car adaptations which can help.

But some problems cannot be helped. Stroke patients may have disturbed vision, a poor appreciation of distance and spatial relationships, poor memory and various other lasting effects which make them dangerous drivers. Sometimes, the stroke patient simply refuses to believe he is no longer fit to drive.

Any stroke patient who wants to drive must notify the authorities of his intention, and have a very thorough checkup with specialists in this area. There are assessment centres with a full range of staff, from driving instructors to opticians. If they say yes, fine. If they say no, then that is final. It can be a very painful moment, and lead to anger and depression. Hopefully, it will in time also lead to a new realism in the patient and free him from dreams which stop him getting in touch with all the things he *can* still do.

Changes in the home

Some months after the stroke, you can finally get a clear idea of how far the patient is likely to progress. Recovery can go on happening for months and years, but it depends on continued therapy, closely tailored to the individual's needs, and continued practice. These may well not be possible, and the potential rewards will rarely be spectacular. Your doctor and therapists will at some point tell you that the patient probably won't recover much more ability.

This is not the end: not at all. It's just that from now on, the emphasis will no longer be on the patient adapting to his environment, but on sizing up the environment and adapting it to what the patient wants to do. Lost functions can still be recovered with the help of small gadgets and aids, and there are many examples of that in this book.

Now it's time to think of major adaptations. If the patient is going to continue to spend a lot of time in a wheelchair, he can be made very independent. We are now talking about very expensive things, so decisions are not to be taken lightly. Major adaptations can often be financed by the state, however. An occupational therapist can, and must, advise on this. You need to be prepared to badger for help if necessary. You need and deserve it, and cannot afford to be put off. Ideas to consider:

- Housing the patient permanently downstairs, and installing a downstairs lavatory and shower unit.
- Ramps to get the wheelchair over small flights of steps (out of the house, for instance).
- Widening doors so a wheelchair can get through them.
- Lowering work surfaces, sinks, kitchen units, etc so the patient can use them.
- Installing a stair lift.
- Getting a better wheelchair, or even two – perhaps a light indoor one, and/or a fold-away one to take on expeditions, and/or a really comfortable adaptable one, and/or a powered model, and/or a rugged outdoor one, and/or a special car and wheelchair system.

FINAL NOTE
One 'major adaptation' might be that the carer gives up caring. You can still care *about* somebody without caring *for* him, day in and day out. No carer should ever be made to think she must carry on no matter what, although other people may be very happy to have her feel that way.

Workbook 4

This whole section is a workbook. Just remember to check it regularly:

- To see if you are still getting all the techniques right.
- To see if the patient is ready for the next step.
- To look back on progress and congratulate each other!

Remember, too, that lifting technique is still important for the carer and her back. Turn back to the lifting advice in section 2 and revise.

And remember that, as the patient gets more independent, the carer must become more independent too. Plan in some time for your own rest, relaxation, friends and interests. A little time is much better than no time at all. But make sure you get it. You need it. It isn't an optional extra.

6

COMMUNICATION

'Problems with communication' is an elegant phrase. What it describes, however, is often hellish. For patients and carers who suffer it, it is the very worst thing about having a stroke.

Solitary confinement has often been used as a form of torture – and with good reason. People are social beings. Losing the power to communicate means boredom, isolation and almost unbearable frustration. But plenty can be done to help.

The vital thing to remember is this. A stroke patient who cannot communicate can still hear. And he is as intelligent as he was before the stroke. He knows he can still think, but he has no way to let other people know it. Carers must do all they can to show him they know it too. Otherwise, he will experience sheer terror. Wouldn't you?

The person who can help is the speech and language therapist, or speech pathologist. She can tell what kind of speech problem the patient has, and knows what to do about it. It is a specialist job. You need expert advice on how to start communicating, and you need it as soon as the patient regains consciousness.

Speech therapists are in very short supply, so treatment may have to stop even when the patient is capable of further progress. The patient may not even be referred to a speech therapist in the first place. Some other professionals believe that it is pointless for stroke patients – especially for those with severe problems.

But, on the contrary, it is the worst cases where the speech therapist can do most. You may have a patient who is left with little or no ability to understand words. He is still as intelligent as ever, and the speech therapist can help you find new ways to communicate.

You may have to nag to get speech therapy. It is almost certainly worth it. If necessary, ask your doctor or nurse how you can get a therapist – and keep asking. If you have to, complain. If all else fails, try to get a speech therapist privately, at least for an initial assessment and some basic advice. But this is a last resort, because it's expensive.

By the way, some people have minor strokes which have no other effect on the body at all – like the lady who was as healthy and as well able to speak as ever, but woke up one morning having lost the ability to add up money. She thought she was going stupid or mad, and became more and more withdrawn until a speech therapist spotted what was really wrong – a tiny stroke which had affected the adding-up part of her brain and nothing else. Well-meaning doctors have been known to administer verbal tests to people who have lost nothing except their fluency with words. Failure to answer properly is marked down as 'mental confusion', but it's the doctor who is confused, not the patient!

The big message is this: focus your energies on breaking down the barriers to communication – NOT on 'curing' the patient's problem. If you (and the other people around) can get some basic know-how in how to communicate, you can make the best of the patient's remaining skills. You can create opportunities for him to communicate. You can, in other words, meet him half-way. Put a patient with someone (however well-meaning) who doesn't know how to do this, and it can be awful. Put the same patient with someone who has these basic skills, and the result is quite different – real communication can take place.

So – the patient may well need speech therapy, and may need to work hard at it. But the person who really needs a bit of 'training' is you! It's by far the easiest (and quickest) way to get communication going.

Don't worry. These skills are really very basic and common sense. And, as someone who knows the patient, you have a head start in working out what he is trying to say!

First, you need to know what the problem is. It could be one of several.

Dysphagia

This is not a speech problem, but it is included in this section because it can sometimes be confused with dysphasia (described in the next part of this section) – and because a speech therapist can help. Dysphagia means an inability to swallow (sometimes, also, inability to chew or suck). Like dysarthria, it is caused by weakness of the throat and mouth muscles.

It is a very unpleasant problem, and not to be treated casually. Since they understand the workings of the muscles involved, speech therapists are often the best professionals to advise. For more on dysphagia, see page 57 in Section 3 (**Early days**).

Dysarthria

The patient can understand language perfectly well, but the stroke has affected the muscles in mouth and throat which control speech. Speech comes out distorted, slurred and drunken-sounding, or may not come out at all. (There may also be problems with swallowing, chewing or breathing because these are controlled by the same muscles.)

These problems usually disappear with time. Speech therapy also helps. It's important to reasssure the patient about this (he can understand you) and encourage him to slow down a bit and be patient. Find other ways to communicate in the meantime, from among the suggestions given in this chapter.

Above all, remember the patient has not lost the power of words. He can still read and understand. With practice, he can write. All that's wrong is weak muscles.

Weak muscles may make a person difficult to understand. They may also sound a little drunk.

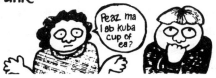

- If you don't understand the patient, say so.
- Dysarthria is worse when the patient is tired.
- You don't need to slow down your own speech, or simplify it, to get through to him. He can understand just as well as he ever did.
- Communication aids can be very helpful. There are all kinds, from flash cards to little electronic communicators. Get advice from a speech therapist.

Dysphasia or aphasia

This is the really tricky one. Here, the patient is neither mad nor stupid – but she has simply lost the ability to understand words, or use them. Sometimes, the patient is also having to cope with dysarthria (page 145) and/or dyspraxia (page 153). In every case, something can be done with the speech therapist's help.

The effects can be mild and annoying (to both patient and carer!), or they can be severe and devastating.

The clinical extent of the problem is not the only factor. One person may be terribly depressed by quite a mild problem. Others keep cheerful even if they have a lot of difficulties. Communication is a very emotional business!

Dysphasia/asphasia happens when the stroke affects the left side of the brain – the side which controls speech and language. (In a very few left-handed people, speech is controlled by the right side of the brain.) About a third of all patients with a stroke will have some degree of dysphasia.

The result: the patient loses some (or all) of her ability to 'de-code' words. She cannot express herself in words. She cannot understand the meaning of words. It is like waking up to find everyone is speaking a foreign language. She can pick up clues from their faces and gestures, but words are useless.

Because it's the language centre of the brain which is affected, people with dysphasia have just as much trouble with reading and writing as they do with speaking and understanding words. In some cases, even pictures don't make much sense until the patient has been shown the objects they represent and learned how to make the connection.

Everyone knows what it is like to misplace a word or a name – to have it 'on the tip of your tongue' and not be able to bring it to mind. For the dysphasic, it feels like that all the time. The frustration is awful. Not surprisingly, the result is often anger or tears. Carers need to understand this, and be patient.

In the first few weeks after the stroke, things will improve spontaneously (at least a little) in all but the worst cases. Spontaneous recovery, at a slower rate, usually goes on for about a year. After that, the only remedy is speech therapy and constant practice. It is very hard work (for the carer, too!), and it can be very tiring.

The most important thing, therefore, is to keep up the patient's morale. The patient has to be encouraged to use whatever communication skills he or she still has. The carer has to learn to pick up every possible signal and, often, to make inspired guesses!

It is not quite as impossible as it seems. One of the fascinating things about dysphasia is finding out what abilities the patient still has. They can be quite surprising. An English aristocrat couldn't say a word – but could play chess as well as ever. A housewife could barely speak – but could sing all the lyrics of a song. A retired nurse found she could still tell the time and deal with numbers. A journalist even found he could manage Latin better than English, and finally made a full recovery.

People who know the patient have a head start in helping. Often, the first words to come back reflect his own special interests – his job, his hobby, family names and so on.

The speech therapist is also trained to spot the abilities which remain, when patient and carer can only see what he *can't* do. She can train you to look out for things to build on. This will make all the difference, and encourage you to press on with finding more and more ways to communicate.

Many stroke patients recover all their ability to communicate – understanding, speaking, reading and writing as well as they ever did. All the same, be prepared for a slow recovery which may never be complete. In general, the more severe the stroke, the worse the problem will be. Sometimes there will be a long period where no progress seems to be made – followed by a sudden 'jump' in communication.

Recent research, however, is starting to prove that progress can still take place years after the stroke. The secret is to work out a programme which suits the individual patient – his needs and his interests, his weak spots and his abilities.

People are very creative. Even a patient who never learns a single word can find other ways to express himself. He can use facial expressions. He can point to things, or build up a stock of useful pictures. He can mime. He can convey a great deal by the tone of his voice.

He may well learn to write a few useful words, or draw pictures. It won't be easy because – of course – a stroke which affects the left side of the brain affects the right side of the body. So he'll probably have the added frustration of learning to use the 'wrong' hand. A typewriter, word processor or other aid may work wonders. He may well learn to read again, although his attention span will be probably shorter.

At the same time, of course, the carer will learn to use the same resources – facial expressions, mime, tone of voice, pictures and so on. One word of caution: people with dysphasia can give out misleading signals, especially in the early stages. They may shake their heads instead of nodding, or say 'yes' instead of 'no'. By using all the expressions at your command, you should be able to sort out quite a workable system. Another word of caution: the way people speak is not a perfect guide to the way people understand. Some people can repeat what you say perfectly – but can't speak for themselves at all. Some people (understandably) pretend to understand, but can't. Some people talk very oddly, or very little, but understand a lot.

And a word of good news: people with dysphasia can often *understand* quite well, even if they can't express themselves. You may be able to say quite a lot, and be understood. You may be able to ask the patient questions to pin down what he means, and get a 'yes' or 'no' signal to tell you if you're on the right track.

For instance, check by asking: 'Are you saying you want more tea?' and point to the tea-pot to give extra help. If you really don't understand, don't pretend you do. If you are both getting really tired, say: 'Let's leave that and try again later.'

One thing you must *not* do is use baby talk, or to talk 'down' to the patient in any way. Use your imagination and realize how frightening, or how maddening, it is to be a perfectly intelligent adult, being addressed like a child or an idiot and not being able to do anything about it!

Another thing you must *not* do is ignore the patient, or talk over his head to other people. Again, it's easy to imagine how hurtful this is, and how miserably isolated it makes the patient feel.

Make sure that family, friends and visitors don't make these two mistakes. You can get leaflets (free, or very cheaply) to explain the basics. Explain, above all, how important it is to keep some kind of communication going – no matter how imperfect it may be. Whatever you do, don't let a communication problem cut you off from friends, family and visitors.

No two cases of dysphasia are alike. This is what makes it so tricky – but also fascinating. To give you an idea, here are four imaginary patients with typical problems. The point, in all cases, is to pick out the things the patient *can* do, and build on them.

Mr A.

Mr A. knows what he wants to say, but can say very little. He just can't find the words. He has trouble understanding, too. Both understanding and talking are very hard work. He may speak in 'telegrams' – just a few key words. He can cope with the meanings of single words, but can easily get into trouble with more complex sentences. He may have more trouble understanding what you say than you at first realize. He may not, for instance, be able to tell the difference between 'The dog is chasing the cat' and 'The cat is chasing the dog'.

He can get his meaning across, but it's hard work for all concerned. He needs to learn to say *more*. See if he's willing to do some reading aloud to get him used to longer sentences. Encourage him to add to his 'vocabulary' by using gestures, drawings, picture cards and so on. Use questions to get him to add to his original 'telegram'. Practise longer and longer sentences. Practise finding lots of words around a common idea (holidays, traffic, hobbies – any topic).

Miss B.

Miss B. knows what she wants to say, and can speak fairly easily. But she often cannot find the right words – especially the names of things. She may use a word similar to the one she wants ('cup' instead of 'plate', for instance), or she may have to find another way round ('thing you sit on' instead of 'chair').

This is all pretty irritating. And the patient will probably be well aware that she is making mistakes, and find the whole business very stressful. She needs lots of encouragement, and lots of practice. Make sure visitors understand what the problem is. Be calm, or humorous, about communication snarl-ups. Encourage communication by all the means available, instead of letting the patient worry about the details that go wrong.

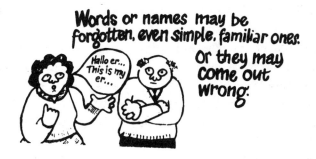

Words or names may be forgotten, even simple, familiar ones. Or they may come out wrong.

Mr C.

Mr C. knows what he wants to say, and can speak fluently. Unfortunately, he has a big problem with understanding. So what comes out may contain lots of real words or even whole phrases ('I'm fine, thank you!') – but the words don't actually reflect what he's trying to say. Or the words might be largely nonsense (sometimes called 'jargon').

For instance, this is a jargon dysphasic's lively description of his job: 'With my jar with the making people and chemical of in this K very echoing the the indoors heavy thing to see where people are.'

He is difficult or impossible to understand, but he has no idea that he is not making sense. This is very irritating, both for the patient and the person trying to get through to him.

He is not helped by rude remarks like: 'Be quiet!' or: 'You're talking rubbish!' He thinks he is making sense, and that you are being stupid or difficult. He needs to learn when people don't understand him — by their questions, facial expressions and so on. Be tactful. Encourage him when he does make sense.

He does need to learn not to go on and on, but this is a delicate matter which needs the speech therapist's advice.

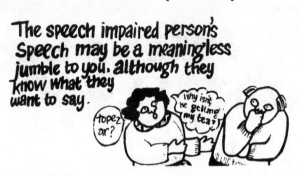

Mrs D.

Mrs D. has very little speech, and very little understanding of words. She may have one or two phrases she uses constantly, whether they fit the situation or not. They may not be real words at all ('la-la-la' or 'beebeep'). This can be quite alarming. They may be real sentences, which are used with no regard to their actual meaning ('It's OK', 'My dear!', 'Why a cat?'). This can be confusing. Swear words are quite common, even in the most respectable of people. This is something you just have to accept, as nicely as you can. Mrs D. doesn't mean to swear, and may be very upset to find herself doing it. All these disconcerting things are absolutely normal in dysphasia.

Mrs D. has the most severe form of dysphasia. In terms of regaining the use of words, very little progress may be made (although some people recover very well indeed). Where words remain hard to use, there's extra incentive to cultivate other forms of communication, from smiles to pictures, from touch to sign language! Get plenty of expert advice.

Remember that morale and motivation are very important. Concentrate on getting some kind of basic communication going right from the start, even if it's just a yes/no signing system. In time, try to master a few important words between you. Remember, above all, that loss of language does *not* mean loss of intelligence. Do all you can to show Mrs D. that you know she is still the same person she always was. And find enjoyable things to do that don't need words (see page 156).

Dyspraxia or apraxia

This is one of the more complicated problems. The speech muscles are not paralysed, but the patient has trouble getting them organized. He simply cannot will them to do what he wants, and what they are physically capable of doing if they are 'taken by surprise'. Licking the lips may be fine, for instance, but deliberate tongue movements to make sounds can be difficult. The more he consciously tries, the more he wills, the worse it works. This makes it very difficult to use speech therapy.

Long words cause more problems than short ones. The problem can be minor, or very severe. Dyspraxia is usually combined with another communication problem (like dysphasia) and can be very difficult and frustrating indeed.

One of the odd things that can happen is that the patient may be able to swear without any problem! Or he may suddenly get out a word clearly when spurred on by anger, or by feeling unusually relaxed. It doesn't mean he could speak at other times, if only he would. It's just one of those baffling things that happens with stroke.

As with dysarthria, the patient with plain dyspraxia/apraxia can usually understand language pretty well. Reading and writing may be easier than speaking. You need to organize other ways to communicate, on the speech therapist's advice. You need to become a very clever listener!

- Progress is slow and variable.
- The patient finds it very hard to correct himself. Trying to imitate other people is no help at all.
- More often than not, people with dyspraxia also have dysphasia.

CLEAR THE GROUND

People with language problems may also have other, quite unrelated, problems which get in the way of communication. So do all you can to get these out of the way.

- The stroke may have caused other problems, such as visual disturbance (especially to the right side) or general disorientation. Check with the professionals and take their advice.
- Make sure the patient is still using any aids he was using before the stroke – like spectacles and dentures. These may need to be replaced by new models.
- Any loss of hearing – even quite trivial – can make understanding much more difficult. Even if the patient didn't need a hearing aid before the stroke, he may benefit from one now (although the stroke has not made hearing worse in itself). Testing for hearing loss is tricky with people who can't communicate, but very worthwhile.

- Drugs may cause problems in communication or make the patient upset or sleepy. Make sure the doctor or pharmacist tells you about any likely side effects, both in drugs prescribed to prevent further strokes and in drugs still being taken for another condition.
- Keep it brief. Stroke survivors don't lose their long-term memory (their life history). But they often lose short-term memory. So they'll get lost in the middle of a long sentence (spoken or written).
- Anxiety and depression are a natural reaction to stroke. It may be possible to treat these with drugs, at least to help things along for a while.
- It is difficult to get your bearings when you're in unfamiliar surroundings. While the patient is still in hospital, take in familiar objects and photographs, well-known visitors and – if possible – pets. If the patient goes into a residential home, do the same.
- Look forward to further progress if the patient can go back to his or her own home. Make as few changes as you can, and surround the patient with familiar objects.
- Establish a routine which is as similar as possible to the patient's old way of life – mealtimes, favourite radio and TV programmes, household tasks.

Small pleasures

People won't feel like trying to communicate if life is not worth living. Sometimes, old pastimes can't be revived so new ones must be found. Your personal knowledge of the patient will help you choose which to try first. All the pleasures listed here are accessible to people with dysphasia. Trial and error is the secret!

- Seat the patient near a window whenever possible, so he can see life going on.
- Set up a bird table to watch, or just a string of nuts to attract birds.
- Consider buying a small pet if you don't already have one – fish, birds or something small and furry in a cage, if you can't face a cat or dog.
- Music is appreciated in the right side of the brain, so a patient with left brain damage can still enjoy it – or discover a new pleasure in it. Use TV, radio, cassettes or records – borrowed from the library if necessary.
- Take the patient outside every day or just to the front door, for a change of scene.
- In the same way, move the patient to a different room at some time, if possible.
- Make sure the patient has access to familiar treasures like jewellery, china and – of course – photographs.
- Buy (or borrow) picture books and magazines on subjects which interest the patient.
- Get him to make a file of magazine clippings (etc) or compile a scrapbook.
- Pay attention to appearance – shaving, hair, make-up, favourite clothes and accessories improve morale. Make sure the patient has a mirror.
- Try painting or colouring (brushes and pens may need to be made thicker and easier to hold by wrapping elastic bands round them).
- See if you can revive interest in an old hobby. But beware – some people find it unbearable to have lost their old skills, and won't want to try.
- Seek out familiar TV and radio programmes – like soap operas, sport or church services – which may revive understanding and pleasure.

- Seek out, too, new TV programmes which don't involve words – sport again, dance, ice skating, nature documentaries, slapstick comedy or mime, circus, educational programmes.
- Jigsaw puzzles can be a pleasant pastime. You may have to start with simple children's puzzles, or make your own by cutting up postcards or clear magazine pictures.
- Be bold and try out all kinds of games to find ones the patient can still play. Chess or draughts may still be possible, and so can card games, like patience, and many board games. Borrow from friends until you find one that clicks.
- Gardening is a good bet – even if it's just a window box, or growing seeds in a jar or tray.

Fight isolation

A language problem is a very lonely thing. Perhaps the most important thing you can do is to make the patient still feel she is a part of things, and can still communicate in some way. This will help to motivate her. Outside visitors are also a boon (for both of you!) – but read the advice in the **Other people** section (page 198). Some people (including children) can't cope at all without some help.

- Touch can convey a strong message, and the initial stress of the stroke may have broken down barriers in people who don't normally touch each other much. Keep up the hugs, kisses and hand squeezes ...
- Make sure the patient has company whenever possible. Bring in small jobs and do them in the patient's room, or just be there reading, knitting or writing. You don't have to talk all the time. (But do remember to give him some privacy, too.)

- Animals are very good at communicating without words. Encourage visitors to bring theirs.
- Babies and small children also make good visitors (but make sure they don't become too tiring).
- Older children can also accept people who can't communicate – often much better than adults. They can sing, put on shows, dress up, show their treasures and toys. People tend to remember best the things they learned early on in life, so nursery rhymes and lullabies may be a big success.
- Children can also be wonderful for playing simple board or card games. An adult stroke patient may find it very hard to play 'childish' games, and feel humiliated by it – but she'll be perfectly willing to indulge a child! She may also be very willing to help them play with their toys and picture books.
- Adult visitors can find it very embarrassing to try to communicate. But they, too, may be able to pass the time agreeably by playing games instead of sitting there trying to talk.
- Adult visitors will also find it easier to communicate if they help the patient carry out a specified task. For ideas, see **Small pleasures** on pages 155–7 and **Suggested tasks** on pages 184–5.
- Don't let any visitor near the patient until she understands the basic do's and don'ts listed under **Basic good manners**.
- Get visitors to make a cup of tea or coffee, or even a light meal, and share it with the patient. This should help cover any gaps in the conversation.
- Encourage visitors to bring things of interest – books, games, records, photographs and so on.

Basic good manners

People with no language are still people, and they need to be treated as such. They can probably understand quite a bit of what you say, and how you are saying it. So you can get a long way just by applying the kind of basic 'good manners' you'd apply with anyone else.

* **Don't** shout. Strokes don't make people deaf.
* **Don't** use baby talk.
* **Don't** ignore the patient or talk over his head. This is very hurtful.
* **Don't** talk about the patient in his presence. He can probably understand you.
* **Don't** finish sentences on the patient's behalf. This is humiliating and frustrating – especially if you get it wrong!
* **Don't** point out, or correct, mistakes the patient makes. He may well be aware of them already, and embarrassed.
* **Don't** cut the patient short rudely if he is talking 'jargon'. He probably thinks he is making perfect sense, and can be easily offended.
* **Don't** lose patience if you can possibly avoid it. A single bad experience can kill the patient's confidence for a long time.
* **Do** try to be positive and enthusiastic. Half-hearted attempts at talk will soon give the patient the message that you don't think it's worth bothering with him.
* **Do** give lots of feedback and support. The patient's self-esteem is very low, and he needs all the encouragement he can get.

Communication checklist

A few basic tips to take the confusion out of communication!

- **Do** try to make sure background noise is at a minimum (eg, turn off the TV).
- **Don't** talk at the same time as other people.
- **Do** make sure the patient knows you are there, knows you want to say something, and can see your face (remember, he may not be aware of things at his paralysed side).
- **Do** speak a little more slowly – but not in a patronizing manner.
- **Do** use just a few words at a time, until you know how much he can take in at one time.
- **Don't** jump quickly from subject to subject. Wait for some reaction from the patient before moving on.
- **Do** give the patient a chance to answer. This takes at least 30 seconds, usually.
- **Do** check you are understood. Most patients can give feedback of some kind, even if it's only a look of puzzlement, distress or boredom!
- **Do** repeat if necessary. Try the same words at first, to give the patient an extra chance to work out your meaning. Then try to convey the same idea, but in different words.
- **Don't** be put off by tears, irritation or other signs of frustration. Put yourself in the patient's shoes for a moment. Surely you can imagine how he feels.
- **Don't** go on and on. Trying to communicate is terribly tiring. Make sure you take a break and just relax together from time to time.

Tips and techniques

- **Don't** assume the patient can understand fully, just because he is smiling or nodding. It may just be good manners, or avoiding the effort of having to understand ...
- **Do** be aware that the patient's words, and even gestures, may not mean what they seem to mean, especially in the early stages of recovery.
- **Do** use other things to back up your own words – gesture, mime, facial expressions, pointing to things, etc – and encourage the patient to do the same.
- **Do** talk about familiar things and people.
- **Do** use questions to try to pin down what the patient is trying to say. Often he can understand and respond, even if he can't say the words himself. Learn to guess!
- **Do** offer choices to respond to. For example, don't say: 'What would you like to drink?' but say 'Would you like tea? Would you like coffee?' (picking up a coffee pot might help, too!).

Communication aids

The success of speech therapy depends on finding an individual solution for each patient, allowing him to make maximum use of the abilities he still has. Sometimes the solution is not to rely solely on words – either spoken or written – but to supplement with whatever body language and visual aids he and the family can conjure up to create their own style of conversation.

Patients who still understand speech can still be reached by giving them a series of questions which they can answer with a 'yes' or 'no' sign. People who know each other well can communicate a lot in this way (if you've ever played '20 Questions' you'll get the idea).

Patients who can understand written language, but cannot control their hands finely enough to write clearly, have a choice of aids to help them, ranging from simple flash cards of useful words to little hand-held mini-computers. A full-scale computer might be very successful.

The speech therapist should advise before any purchase is made. The wrong aid is worse than no aid at all. Bear in mind that, as physical handicaps get better, more things become possible. One man progressed from blinking once for 'yes' and twice for 'no', to tapping out a code, to using a gadget with big buttons for his clumsy fingers, to using a sophisticated keyboard. His understanding of words was always fine – but his body skills had to catch up.

For patients who cannot understand words, or can understand very few, there are still many possibilities. Body language and gesture, of course, come into their own. There are picture flash cards of common objects, picture dictionaries and small electronic aids which help translate pictures into words in other ways. Again, the speech therapist should advise.

Another possibility is sign language. One example is Amerind, originally developed by North American Indians so that different tribes could talk together. The signs are so clear that most people can understand them without having them explained, although newly-created words can be a bit clumsy. Instead of miming 'water' and 'seat' for 'lavatory', it might be quicker just to make a chain-pulling movement, for instance. But quite elaborate conversations can be carried out.

Practice makes perfect

Perfecting a new language – verbal or otherwise – takes patience and practice. Carer, visitors and family will almost certainly find themselves helping the speech therapist's work between sessions. It is very important to get her advice on what to do. Any attempt to communicate is better than none, but its effects will be so much more successful if you know what you are doing, and what the patient has been learning to do with the therapist. Ask to attend some sessions (the therapist will want to work alone with the patient at least some of the time).

What you *must* get clear in your mind is exactly what the patient can and cannot do. Otherwise your attempts to communicate will be destined to fail, and the patient will be humiliated and frustrated for no reason. This is exactly how best to discourage him.

So ask a speech therapist to explain the patient's ability in the four main functions of language: understanding the written word; understanding the spoken word; writing, speaking. Some people can understand very well, but cannot speak or write purely because of weak muscles in throat or hand. Other people can understand, cannot speak because of weak muscles, but can write because their hands are all right. Others have limited understanding. Others again cannot understand words at all – so they can neither speak nor write even if their mouth and hand muscles are fine. Find out where your particular patient stands. Communicate with him accordingly, and make sure visitors also understand the basics.

You now have a range of interlocking skills, all at different levels, all of them needing practice at the right level. Handbooks of games for practice are published, and you can supplement these with games recommended by the speech therapist. But you do need her guidance in picking out the set of skills which your particular patient needs to master, and the games which will develop them.

The possibilities are endless, from question and answer games, to picture matching games like 'snap' and dominoes, from copying words and drawings to reading aloud. Once you have the basic personalized advice you need, a host of activities will be possible. But beware – if the game seems childish, some people will find it humiliating and upsetting.

And don't forget the surprising abilities which even severely dysphasic patients may retain. Many can sing when they can't talk. Games, from draughts through to chess, may be played with as much skill and enjoyment as ever. One man could even follow the stock market, although he had great difficulty remembering his own name. Experiment, with tact and patience, and see what you find. Such pastimes are precious to people with no speech: for once, they are communicating on the same level as everyone else.

Make every effort to get a dysphasic patient into a stroke club or, even better, a specialist speech club where dysphasic people can socialize and practise. Again, such clubs are precious because the patient is on the same level as everyone else – and may well encounter people with even worse problems than his own.

Learning to communicate, then, takes ingenuity. It also takes great patience, great tact, and unswerving respect for the patient's dignity. Not being able to speak is the most frustrating and embarrassing of all the disabilities which are caused by stroke.

Don't be put off by crying, irritation or other signs of frustration. Sometimes these feelings must be acknowledged, and need to be expressed. But if they happen often it may be best to ignore them, or change the subject. They may just indicate tiredness and the need to rest from attempting communication. At other times encouragement to continue may be the right response. Professional advice may be useful, but so may your own sensitivity and knowledge of the person. A stroke causes some people to cry or laugh when they don't mean it. Ignoring this helps them to get these feelings under control more quickly.

For some, being taught to speak is the last straw. They can cope psychologically with learning to walk again, and may not mind being instructed by a close relative – but being taught to speak by the same person is intolerable. Take advice from the speech therapist again, and perhaps you can delegate this particular task to somebody else (it is, after all, an interesting task if you know what you are doing and why).

A really good idea is to find out if there is a local group or club for people with dysphasia (see **Clubs**, page 233).

Every stroke patient can learn to communicate again, in one way or another. And he must. Nothing is more essential to his quality of life – and nothing is more rewarding, to patient, carer, friends and family!

Occasionally someone may reject speech therapy altogether. They may simply not be ready to accept the reality of what has happened and may believe that they are going to wake up better one day. If the speech and language therapist tells you that your relative is not benefiting from therapy, try to find out if this attitude is the cause. It is not uncommon for someone to be much more receptive after some time has elapsed and they have come to terms with what has happened to them.

Don't give up hope

If you are stuck for words after a long time, it's worth seeing what a reassessment of the problems may do. A new idea may come up which can finally break down the barriers. Miracles are rare, but it's slowly being proved that today's therapists can achieve results which were thought impossible a few years ago – and are still thought impossible by some people you may encounter.

The final word, then, goes to a stroke patient's own progress report:

> *I thought I will write and let other people know what has happen to me after a stroke.*
>
> *It happen at tea-time on the 3rd February 1987. I could not talk, and the doctor came to see me and siad it was a stroke and that he would see me again in two or three days. He siad to my wife isn't it a shame, meaning my not able to speake.*
>
> *The next move was to go and see the speech therapist. That was the best thing to happen to me. I then made up my mind I was determined I will talk popley agian. So the fight was on. And I noticed each day I say a few more words.*
>
> *About the 20th April I went to see the doctor again. And he siad to me that I would not speake much better than I do now, I belive my vocabulary was only 15%.*
>
> *Beginning of May the next move. The speech therapist asks me if I would like to join her speech class along with other patients. This done wodners for me.*
>
> *Today my vocabulary is 90% plus and I belive I will talk 100% eventually.*
>
> *My belive if you can fight you will succeed. I am still fighting.*

The writer has since completely regained the ability to write, with perfect spelling, and he is now working on articles for magazines. A lot of people don't get this far, but do learn to communicate everything they want to say ...

Workbook 5

This whole section is full of lists of suggested actions. Go back through it regularly and check:

- that you are still carrying out all the details, and haven't forgotten any
- that you really know how to explain to visitors what to do, and why
- that you can now try something you couldn't do before
- that a new problem you have just noticed might be explained somewhere in the beginning of the section.

You can use care planning to help you list and carry out your choice of the actions suggested – and to identify any small problems that stand in your way. Do things in small, easy steps – the easiest one first.

Celebrate any success – however small.

Make sure everyone knows about any new way you have found to communicate, so they can all use it.

Ask a speech and language therapist or speech pathologist for advice on other things you can do to increase communication. There is an enormous choice of games to play and things to do – all working on quite different speech problems. So you need expert advice to be sure you are using the best ones for your particular patient.

7

DAILY LIVING

This section widens the focus. So far, much of the book has concentrated on the vital early tasks of nursing, rehabilitation and (for those who need to do it) learning to communicate. It's important to get these right and to start them as soon as possible, or the patient's long-term quality of recovery is in danger. They have to take priority. But what happens next?

Some patients get very rapidly through the dependent state and are soon back to normal with very little help. Some patients will have to work long and hard to win back the same level of independence. People with severe strokes will never be able to do all the things they did before. For them, maximum recovery means working out a lifestyle – perhaps in a wheelchair, perhaps with no language – which is as near as possible to normal, and as enjoyable to live as possible, and puts as little strain as possible on the carer.

Finally, there will be patients who cling stubbornly to the dependent state, when professional advisers tell you they could easily do more. There are many possible reasons for this: shattered confidence, shattered self-image, depression, fear that the carer will leave if she gets the chance, enjoyment of a suddenly acquired power to dominate other people's lives. Getting them to co-operate will be a psychological as well as a physical battle.

You can start using the ideas in the section as soon as you like. With some patients, you will succeed at once and can progress rapidly through the whole section, with the patient taking over more and more control and the carer steadily bowing out. Other patients will never get to the end of the section.

At the time you start, there will be no way of knowing how full the patient's recovery is going to be. So use this section flexibly. Flip through and try whatever ideas patient and carer most fancy. These are the ones which are most likely to work.

And use it with a very selective eye. Don't try to do too much, all at the same time. The patient may hate being 'babied' and be anxious to get back in control. The carer, of course, needs to off-load as much work as possible, as soon as possible. But be warned.

Even simple skills will have to be laboriously re-learned, sometimes with the 'wrong' hand, and problems with vision and touch can make things desperately difficult. You need to understand what these problems are, for your particular patient, or his behaviour can look infuriatingly stupid. Whatever the stroke has done to him, it has *not* made him stupid.

It is all too easy, too, to accuse the patient of not trying, or of being lazy. Sometimes, of course, he *is* being uncooperative and lazy. You need proper knowledge of his physical and sensory problems to be able to tell whether you're up against a practical problem or a problem with motivation and morale.

First efforts are almost guaranteed to be infuriating all round. Infuriating for him because everything is so difficult; infuriating for you because he is so slow. It's the carer who has to make the concessions here. It may be infinitely quicker to do the task yourself, but if you don't put up with this you may end up doing all the work, all the time, and have a very dependent and demoralized patient.

Carers will need to call on all their patience. Getting annoyed with the patient will wreck his self-esteem and make him less keen to go on trying. Break down each task into *very* small steps, which are almost sure to be successful. And when there is a success, make sure it is pointed out and praised. You can do this without being patronizing if you have a grasp of what the difficulties are.

Let the patient do things in his own time. If he is not put under stress by being hurried up, he will do better. And make sure he has plenty of rest between tasks. Above all, steel yourself to cope with tears, anger and other signs of frustration. It will all pay off in the end.

Planning

Whatever the task in hand, you'll need planning skills to get the patient doing it. The basics are the same as for care planning: small, precise goals which highlight small successes and build up, step by step, into complete plans of action.

You will need to work out what equipment is needed, whether it's the patient's comb and mirror or the full panoply of water, bowl, washing up liquid, dishcloth and waterproof sheet needed to cope with washing the dishes. In time, you will make sure the patient can get hold of these things for himself, by putting them in an accessible drawer or cupboard.

You may need to change the places where you keep things, and keep related equipment all together. Low storage spaces are a boon for those still spending most of their time in chairs or wheelchairs – maybe someone could put in some extra low shelves, or some accessible wall hooks.

The eventual aim will be to enable the patient to do the whole job himself. Certain routines (like feeding the cat) should be done at regular times, without prompting. For patients who have problems with memory, concentration or simply telling the time, this will be a very major achievement, and may be too high to aim at with any realism. But do try. You may be pleasantly surprised.

To get started, you need the analytical skills of an occupational therapist. With her advice, you can learn to pick out all the functions – mental and physical – which have to be mastered in order to do a task. Then you have to find your own ways round the obstacles. This calls for a blend of ingenuity and sheer common sense. Often, a visitor will come up with a solution you were too involved to see yourself. Trying will certainly make for some interesting conversations!

ROUTINE FOR LIVING
Getting organized is your basic tool for easing back into a normal, workable lifestyle. For some people, the whole idea of a routine is rather depressing – but it really does pay off, especially in the early days.

The patient needs to feel secure. He may find it very difficult to think what to do next, and to make even simple decisions such as when to have a bath. A routine helps overcome these problems, and speeds his progress towards feeling more in control of things.

Carers also need to know where they are. Establishing habits will lessen the general feeling of chaos and panic. It will also help the patient become more independent, and help establish a few ground rules about what the carer is – and is not – prepared to contribute. Carers must plan in their own needs, right from the start, so they don't get dragged into a patient-centred lifestyle in which they have no sense of independence or identity.

Having a routine – written down – also makes it easier to check that both patient and carer are achieving a balanced, satisfying lifestyle which includes: useful work, enjoyable leisure, rest, privacy, social contact and getting out of the house. If these aims are kept firmly in mind, there's no reason why even the most handicapped patient or the busiest carer can't manage them. If there are problems in any of these areas, you will be able to identify them and think about solutions.

- Build up a weekly schedule which includes: housework (Monday washing, Tuesday ironing, Wednesday shopping and so on), appointments (therapy, weekly club, day centre etc), TV programmes, outings (church, a drive, visits). At least one 'major event' per day!
- Build up a daily schedule which includes: getting up and dressing, preparing meals and clearing them up, therapy activities, rest periods, possibly trips to the lavatory, feeding pets, possibly medication. All at regular times.
- Remember to spread the patient's limited energy throughout the day. Getting dressed, for instance, is time-consuming, physically tiring and may be intellectually tiring too. So build in a rest period afterwards if it's needed.
- In the same way, you may need to build in a rest period *before* a demanding activity such as an outing, or entertaining guests (especially small children!) If this

is neglected, well-meant treats may turn into emotional disasters!

- Realize that therapy work is often frustrating as well as exhausting. Plan short, frequent sessions. Tiredness and upset leads to failure – which destroys the patient's self-esteem and willingness to try again.

Keep a diary

Once you have some kind of daily and weekly routine, write it out clearly and make it into a daily record. This is especially useful if the patient has language problems, is depressed, lacks motivation, is confused or has a poor memory. Many of these afflictions, of course, apply to carers as well!

The diary could become something of a scrapbook, containing postcards and letters received, interesting pictures and oddments, messages from visitors, helpers and professionals. It can be the patient's task to stick things in, keep it in order and invite people to contribute.

It can also become a very important working tool:

- It is a genuinely important job for the patient – and a responsibility.
- The patient can keep it by him, to help him keep track of what is happening.
- It may save the carer from repeating certain bits of information over and over again.
- It becomes very useful to show to visitors and helpers, so they know what to do.
- Similarly, a record of who's visited and what has been happening is very useful in starting a conversation.
- It can be used by professionals to record new tasks, methods to be used and targets.

- Visitors and helpers can record what they have done, so their efforts are co-ordinated.
- It can build up a useful checklist of who does what with the patient, what topics of conversation are successful, what activities turn out to be enjoyable for both.
- If the diary is frank enough – and why shouldn't it be? – it can also record upsets, which will help both patients and carers be aware of the effects they have on each other.
- This can be built on to pinpoint events or remarks which trigger these upsets, so both patient and carer can identify the real problems – and experiment with solutions.
- It can identify problems which an outside visitor might be able to solve.
- The diary can record breakthroughs – new ways of communicating, new activities – so that everyone is up to date and able to take advantage.
- It can be a source of bright ideas when nobody can think of anything to do.
- Most important of all, the diary must record successes – however small. This boosts morale all round by making sure these successes are properly registered. And it can be good to look back on past successes when progress seems slow.
- Records of past successes may even furnish ideas to help with current problems. Ingenuity can sometimes run low, especially in patient and carer, who are too close to stand back and see things clearly, or are just plain tired or jaded.

Aids to help you

There are many simple gadgets which make awkward jobs easier for ordinary people – never mind disabled people. They can make all the difference between success and failure. But don't get carried away.

- Beware of using an aid for everything. The patient may become dependent on it, when in time he could have learned to do the job without it. Aids should help rehabilitation – not block it.
- Avoid ugly, clinical-looking aids if you can. Stroke patients are not ill, and their confidence and self-image can be damaged. On the other hand, such aids are the most likely to be available free of charge, so watch your budget.
- You don't necessarily need a special gadget 'for the disabled'. They may be expensive – and tests by British occupational therapists show they are often very poorly designed. Ordinary 'consumer' versions often exist, and actually work better.
- Remember that each aid has to be suitable for the individual who will use it. Every patient has different skills, and there is often a range of similar aids to choose between.
- Get as much information as you can. Ask an occupational therapist, swap notes with other carers, browse through catalogues.
- If you possibly can, try before you buy. You may be able to borrow an aid to test it, or buy larger aids on approval.
- Never spend money on major aids until several months have passed and you have been told the patient is

unlikely to make much further progress. That's when you'll know what you really need. Remember, aids and clever techniques will enable the patient to do more and more, even when his functional ability remains static.

- From time to time, review the aids the patient is using. Does he still really need them all? Has a confidence-booster turned into a dependency-creator?

The lavatory

Most people are keen to look after themselves in this department, even before they can stand up or walk. Carers, too, will probably have this high on their list of tasks they would like to unload!

- The first step is for the patient to handle his or her own urinal or bottle in bed.
- Equally important is for the patient to take charge of wiping with toilet paper.
- The next step might be to use a bottle or urinal when sitting on the bed or (safer) a chair.
- Another idea is a commode in the patient's own room. You may well be able to get one on loan – you'll hope to be able to do without it in the end. If the patient has to be helped to the commode it is, of course, highly desirable to leave him in privacy until he has finished.
- Once he can get to the lavatory, everyone will be much happier. In the early days, try to ensure the door opens outwards, so you can get in if he falls.
- A raised lavatory seat makes getting on and off much easier. You can get one which can be removed easily by other members of the family. If the extra height leaves the patient's legs dangling, add a sturdy, stable footstool.

- Grab rails are probably essential – either attached (firmly!) to the wall, or a free-standing frame-like unit (some of them can be folded away).
- Bear in mind that men have extra problems as most will prefer to stand up to urinate, as they always have, so they may need extra supporting rails. They might like to start off by using a bottle over the lavatory, in case their aim is not very good. They can do this with one hand, and balance against the carer or – better still – the wall.
- Check that the patient can reach the toilet paper holder and the lavatory chain or handle. But check, also, that they won't be used as extra grab rails – they will probably break.
- Tearing sheets from a roll of toilet paper is a two-handed job! Use a brand which dispenses single sheets.
- There are many, many other aids to using the lavatory. If the simple ones outlined here don't work well enough, find out what else you can get.

Keeping clean

A wash or a bath is a pleasure as well as a task – and all the better if you can do it alone. Most patients should be motivated to learn to look after themselves.

- Start with a bowl of water in the patient's room – on a good, solid surface and with a non-slip mat underneath. Put a towel on the chair before the patient sits down.
- Encourage the patient to hold the flannel or sponge in his weak hand right from the start, guiding it with his strong hand until he no longer needs to do so.

- Once in the bathroom, a chair in front of the washbasin is a good idea until the patient has the confidence and energy to stand up and keep his balance.
- Be very safety-conscious in the bathroom – non-slip mats, non-slip stickers in the bath, an eagle eye for clutter.
- Put one or two well-placed grab rails round washbasin and bath.
- Long-handled bath brushes, sponges and loofahs make it easier to reach the whole body.
- Soap on a rope, attached to something strong, stops soap flying out of reach.
- Lever handles on taps make them much easier to turn.
- Getting into the bath is a major undertaking. There are many bath-boards or bath seats which the patient can get on to (even from a wheelchair, with help).
- Showers are invaluable – anything from a simple rubber attachment to put on the taps, to a plumbed-in shower unit (you can get special shower stools, rather like a lavatory seat on legs, so that the patient can sit securely and still reach everything he wants to wash).
- Much cheaper, and still effective, is a plastic bidet which can be placed on the lavatory and filled with water.
- Some precautions when using the bath: don't let in the hot water first, just in case the patient falls in and scalds himself; don't put the affected arm or leg into the water first – if it's too hot, the patient may not feel this; let out the bath water before the patient gets out.
- There are many, many other aids to washing and bathing. If the simple ideas outlined here don't work, find out what else is available.

Food and drink

For most people, these are great pleasures. Stroke patients need all the enjoyment they can get. They are *not* likely to enjoy being fed by another person – few things can be more humiliating, and few things are more likely to encourage the feeling of being a dependent invalid.

From the carer's point of view, feeding is a task to be off-loaded as soon as possible. It can keep the patient occupied for quite some time, and leave her in peace to have her own meal. Carers need to care for their own health.

- A few cheap gadgets can make eating very much easier – non-slip mats to go under plates, non-slip eggcups, specially designed cutlery (including one-handed and large-handled versions), specially designed plates with sloping bottoms to help scoop up food, plate guards to fix round ordinary plates for the same purpose.
- Some rather more expensive gadgets do the same jobs but look much more attractive. The investment might do wonders for morale.
- Baby equipment (bought or borrowed) can be useful – in particular, plates with a hot water compartment to keep food hot when eating is slow and difficult. But try to avoid nursery patterns, unless the patient has a good sense of humour!
- There will be problems with patients who have lost one side of their vision. They simply don't know there is food on one side of the plate. Point it out, or move the plate round.
- Meals should be small and frequent.
- Don't be upset if the patient has lost his taste for old favourites. Altered sensations can have this effect.

- Do make sure the patient gets plenty to drink.
- Do make sure the patient's meals have plenty of protein, preferably low fat (eggs, fish, meat, beans, low fat milk, cheese and yoghurt) and vitamin C (tomatoes, oranges, cherries and potatoes are good sources). Both these help to heal and rebuild damaged tissue.
- Do make sure the patient's meals are high in fibre (beans and peas, whole grain bread, rice, cereal, pasta, added-bran foods and – less useful – fruit and vegetables). Constipation is bad for health and bad for morale.
- Do, despite all this advice, have simple meals regularly. 'Something on toast' can be as nutritious as something more elaborate – and carers need to guard against working too hard all the time.
- Do, if you're a carer, pay as much attention to your own diet as the patient's. Your own health matters – very much.
- There's no reason to deny the patient alcohol, although excessive drinking can only make his problems worse.

Getting dressed

Getting dressed in quite complicated. Patients will have special problems if they have to use the 'wrong hand', or mainly one hand, or have problems with vision or sensory loss. People with ataxia (lack of coordination) or apraxia (inability to do things at will) will need to practise and practise for even a small chance of success.

Carers will probably spend a long time helping the patient before they can leave him alone to do the whole task. And it will probably tire him out. But these ideas will help:

- Make sure the room is warm, so speed isn't vital.
- Arrange garments in a pile, in the order they will be put on.
- Store garments in exactly the same place and order every time, so the patient can learn to get them out himself.
- Always use exactly the same method for dressing, so the patient learns it (the basic methods are outlined in Section 3 – **Early days**).
- Do as much dressing as possible sitting down.
- Have a footstool to help with shoes and socks.
- Regard 'dressing aids' with suspicion, as they are often almost useless. Try before you buy – especially stocking aids.
- Two good ideas – a long-handled shoe horn and a floor-mounted shoe jack.
- Home-made aid worth trying – an old wooden coat-hanger, hook removed, preferably with a rubber thimble over one end for a better grip. Use it to hook stray straps over shoulders.
- Harder to manage, but cheap enough to try – a hook and string device to catch a zip and pull it up.

Clothes

Lack of balance, and awkward fingers, can make dressing difficult. Sensory, visual and mental problems can make it almost impossible without constant supervision. Awkward clothes, however, are a quite unnecessary nuisance. It is hardly ever necessary to buy special clothes 'for the disabled', and such garments can be dreary and demoralizing.

Instead, bear some simple ideas in mind when you're going through an existing wardrobe of clothes – or shopping (or hinting) for new ones.

- garments which fasten at the front (including bras)
- garments which have no fastenings at all (blouses, T-shirts, dresses, sweaters)
- casual wear, like tracksuits (these can look good even on a 90-year-old!)
- elasticated waists (put them in pyjamas, too)
- cardigans, if sweaters are awkward
- wide necks and arms
- hold-up stockings or single-leg tights
- large buttons
- zip or Velcro fastenings (the latter simply stick together, and are easily sewn to existing garments and even shoes)
- slip-on shoes
- elasticated shoelaces, which turn lace-ups into slip-ons
- clip-on ties
- aprons with a sprung waistband – they can be slipped on and don't need tying
- wrap-around skirts
- really smart housecoats and dressing gowns for times when getting dressed is more than patient or carer can face
- stretchy fabric with lots of 'give' for manoeuvring
- loose-fitting clothes of all kinds
- clothes with pockets (especially for people who need handkerchiefs for dribbling etc and forgetful people).

If incontinence continues to be a problem after the first few days, clothes will become a major aspect of your plans to deal with it. Some of the ideas above will be specially useful in enabling hasty access to the loo or commode, such as elasticated trousers, wrap-around skirts (put the wrap-over at the back), and single-leg tights.

Other useful devices, of particular relevance to incontinence, include: French knickers and split-crotch versions (pretty ones can be found in ordinary shops) which don't have to be pulled down to be got out of the way; adaptations for trousers (including a longer fly, to accommodate a urinal, and front or back flaps secured by Velcro) and clothes adapted to conceal the bag for a long-term urinary catheter. Incontinence is a specialized subject, so seek specialist advice on managing it.

Being useful

So far, we have concentrated on the personal tasks of daily living. They are the ones which, usually, patients are keenest to take over and carers are keenest to stop doing.

But they do tend to focus the patient's attention inwards on herself. Some stroke patients become very self-centred, and seem to care nothing about anyone else. Even if this isn't the case, the patient has too much time to brood and be introspective. She needs to have her eyes focused on something beyond her own navel.

The patient badly needs some kind of purpose in life. She needs to feel she's not completely without value. So she can benefit from having something to do which is genuinely useful, and for which she can be given genuine responsibility.

The obvious place to look for ideas is within the household. Below are some suggestions, starting with one or two very simple ones which can be done by people who are still pretty confused. Once you start looking around, you will doubtless spot plenty more for yourselves.

Be sensitive about the choice of task. It must ideally be something the patient wants to do, or at least is willing to do – although a little bullying may be called for with a patient who clings to her helplessness.

Men, especially elderly men, may not take kindly to doing housework, although some tasks will be more acceptable than others. Women, equally, can be very upset by their poor skills, in an area which they used to manage with ease.

Three things can help. First is a sense of humour! Second is the strong awareness most patients have that their stroke has created an enormous amount of worry and work for the carer. They will want to help out if they can.

Third is visitors. Instead of sitting and trying to make bright conversation, they can sit with the patient and tackle one of these tasks together, sharing their problem-solving skills. Male visitors, in particular, might be scared stiff of having to comfort an invalid (as they see it) and will enjoy exercising their ingenuity. With luck, they may even be drawn into making simple aids or adaptations!

The ultimate morale booster might be for an outsider to bring in a task. Does the patient's old club have a jumble of photographs to be mounted? Would the neighbours like their silver polished? Can your niece bring in that Afghan hound which needs regular brushing? Start looking for ideas and you never know what you might find.

Suggested tasks

- help to wind wool
- unravel knitting or knots
- sort things out – pairs of socks, untidy shelves and cupboards, books, old photographs, cutlery tray
- dust
- clean silver, or shoes (messy, but not hard to do one-handed)
- feed birds, goldfish, other pets

- brush pets
- brush people's hair
- set the table
- wash or dry dishes – perfectly possible with one hand
- wash small items of clothing
- peel and chop fruit and vegetables – secure them on a spiked board
- cut bread or cake – ditto
- beat eggs, cake mixes
- make pastry and crumble mix
- open the post
- change the calendar
- wind clocks and watches

The kitchen

In many households, the kitchen is a focus of family life, and that family life should include the patient. It is also a major working area, and the carer is likely to spend quite a lot of time there. Having the patient with her saves worry and constant scuttling back and forth to another room.

The patient can sit quietly and watch the comings and goings. But he or she can also find plenty of small tasks to do. In time, he can cook full-scale meals if the stroke has not made him too forgetful to be safe, or too impaired in judgment to devise edible meals.

Meantime, there are plenty of jobs to be done. The ultimate target is to enable the patient to pursue a single task from start to finish without help, from taking out the things he needs to putting them all back again. The trick is to have an organized kitchen:

- Store the same things in the same place, in the same order, all the time.
- Store together things which are used together (for instance, kettle, coffee, sugar, spoons, cups, saucers).
- Use the same crockery every day for the different meals (for instance, blue cups means it's breakfast!).
- Make better use of low cupboards, easily reached from chair or wheelchair, to store things the patient is likely to use.
- Label things. This is especially useful for patients who are learning to read again, and also makes it much easier to rope in visitors to help, without having to explain where everything is all the time.
- Install some low shelves, or hooks low on the wall.
- Squeeze in a low, solid table or trolley if you can, for the patient to work at.

Many useful aids can be home-made, using ordinary common sense. The most important thing to check is that they are stable and secure. Safety is the most important consideration, and there are many devices to protect small children which you can take advantage of. Other small aids can be bought very cheaply, often in ordinary houseware shops. Here are some ideas:

- a secure tip-up base to take the kettle, tea-pot and coffee-pot, so the patient can pour without having to lift it up
- a spiked board to hold fruit and vegetables secure while they are peeled and chopped
- a breadboard with two pieces of beading nailed down at right angles, to hold the bread steady while it is cut
- a secure base to hold mixing bowls

- non-slip mats, for just about anything (alternative – a damp cloth)
- devices for unscrewing awkward jars (from simple rubber grips to wall-mounted devices)
- a wall-mounted tin opener
- large, easy to read and handle controls for the cooker
- lever taps/faucets for the sink
- a small vice, mounted at the table edge, which can adjust to hold things tightly
- electrically operated knives and similar labour-saving gadgets
- saucepans with magnetic feet which stay firm on the cooker while the contents are stirred
- something to gather up dangling flexes
- electric plugs with large handles
- one-handed knives which work by rocking rather than sawing (make sure the patient uses the other hand to steady the work, if he can do it safely)
- guards to stop pans being tipped over by the handles
- a fire guard to protect the oven door – many ovens are scaldingly hot on the outside
- unbreakable dishes – attractive ones should be easy to find
- an anti-splatter cover for the frying pan
- long-handled or extendable tongs to pick up dropped objects
- a wire basket to fit inside saucepans, so cooked items can be easily lifted out and drained

Leisure

The one thing a stroke is liable to add to your life is time. For a formerly busy person, this is a torment in itself. The carer, too, can feel the same frustrations. Both may be confined indoors much more than before. Both may not be able to concentrate on reading – the carer can't relax for long enough; the patient may have trouble reading, or remembering what he has read.

For both these people, leisure activity is not a luxury but an absolute necessity for sanity. Both need to focus on what they can do, rather than on what they can no longer do. Both need time away from each other, and a chance to maintain separate interests and identities. Both will probably find there is nothing quite as good as getting right out of the house – and doing it without the carer/patient at least some of the time.

Almost anything can become a new and satisfying leisure pursuit. There is space here only for a few ideas. But there are two basic strategies. One is to maintain old interests, which helps counter the feeling that life has completely changed – for the worse. Often a few well-chosen aids can allow the activity to continue almost as before. Sometimes, you need to 'scale down' the activity: if you used to play a sport, for instance, you may still enjoy watching it or looking at relevant books.

The second strategy is to find something new. Often, there is something which has always interested you but could not be fitted into your lifestyle. The most useful possibilities are quiet indoor pursuits, and excuses for outings and visits. A new interest is the strongest possible proof that life – either for patient or carer – did not come to an end with the stroke.

Word processor

This is much easier to handle than a typewriter, and there are many small aids and adaptations to make it even easier. Many stroke patients, and carers, have discovered a taste and a talent for writing – from letters to full-scale novels.

Computer

Here, the possibilities are almost endless, from tie-ins with international data banks to sophisticated computer graphics. The main limit, of course, is finance. But quite a lot of fun can be got out of a cheap domestic or even children's model – especially for dysphasic patients. Older people, who would never otherwise have gone near a computer, may surprise themselves with their computer skills.

Painting and sketching

Again, many aids can be used. It may well be hard work to control a pen or brush, but the results will be more successful than attempts at writing. Abstract patterns, with lots of colour, can substitute for attempts at realistic drawing.

Music

This is a pleasure accessible to the most handicapped – even those who have lost all language. Headphones can help prevent driving other people mad. Make a point of expanding your tastes – borrow cassettes and records from friends or a library to see what you might have been missing.

Gardening

Useful aids can often be bought at an ordinary garden centre, and include long-handled and/or lightweight tools of all kinds. Raised flower beds can make all the difference or, failing that, tubs. And don't forget window boxes and indoor plants.

Talking on the phone

Again, you won't need specialized aids now that telephones come with remote control amplifiers, push button dialling, hands-off holders and so on. For basic messages (and emergencies) you can get a phone that plays recorded messages for someone who can't speak.

Study

If you can read, there are all kinds of correspondence courses from hobby level to degree level. You might even learn some skills which could earn money ... You can also – at last! – take advantage of educational programmes on TV and radio. As soon as the patient can get into a wheelchair, and provided the relevant buildings have wheelchair access, there are the library, the museum, the art gallery, the local college and evening classes. Many, these days, have programmes to cater for all kinds of disabilities.

Craft work

This might smack of 'basket weaving to keep the patient occupied', but there is such a range of possibilities that something can be found which is interesting and at the right level of ability. Carers may well find they can settle down to craft work when they can't relax into anything else.

Talking books

When reading is tiring or impossible, patients who can understand speech can borrow a range of talking books which they can switch on or off to suit their attention span. Family letters could be sent in cassette form, too.

Chess, bridge etc

Games like this are intellectually deeply absorbing, and they can be miraculously accessible to patients without language. At a simpler level, many people can still enjoy card games, children's games like snap and dominoes, and board games like draughts or checkers. There are ingenious aids, including: playing card holders, extra large cards and large pieces for board games. Solo games like patience and solitaire are especially valuable for giving patient and carer a break from each other.

Sports

Even wheelchair-bound and severely handicapped people can still play sport if they can summon the heart for it – or be pushed into it. Swimming is a particularly good bet, while special organizations provide advice, aids and events for disabled competitors. Think of a sport and find out what's possible. And don't forget spectator sports. Physical activity is very good for stress – carers please note!

Clubs

Clubs are mentioned elsewhere, but must be included in any leisure list. They fall into two groups: clubs which have something to do with stroke, disability or caring (valuable for swapping notes with people who understand), and clubs which have nothing to do with disability (valuable for remembering you are a whole human being). Patients and carers have equal need for both of these things.

Holidays

Many holiday places can accommodate disabled people, with or without their carers. If the patient can't possibly get away, or adamantly refuses to do so, the carer has every justification for getting away herself at least once a year. She should move heaven and earth to do so. One word of caution: take advice on holiday venues from experts on disability. Commercial hotels (etc) sometimes mean well when they offer special facilities, but they often don't have a clue what's really needed.

Getting out

Above all, both patient and carer *must* aim to get out of the house every day, even if it's only a wheelchair run to the shops (supermarkets have lots of space and won't try to hurry you up) or into the garden. Four walls close in on the happiest person, and lack of daylight can be a cause of depression.

Sex

Many elderly stroke patients gave up sex years ago. From a modern point of view this is a tragedy, but it's the patient and spouse's choice. Other elderly people have had no such inhibitions, and deserve as much help in reviving their sex life as anyone else. Younger people are likely to show the same variations in previous activity.

Wild guesses are not in order. Probing questions take away dignity. All the same, there's room for sensitive awareness that there may be problems, and a need to get some facts straight.

First, strokes very seldom take away a man's sexual potency. The problems, if any, are much more likely to be psychological – and, of course, all the more tricky for that. In this respect, male stroke patients are just the same as other men.

Second, sex is very unlikely indeed to bring on a second

stroke — a major, and often unvoiced, fear for stroke patient and spouse. A possible exception to this rule is when the stroke was caused by a cerebral haemorrhage. A sharp rise in blood pressure may bring on another haemorrhage, and blood pressure does rise sharply at orgasm. Sexual excitement short of orgasm is much better than nothing if there really is a risk.

You need advice from your doctor about the nature of the patient's stroke and whether there's a risk. To repeat — such a risk is rare. If the doctor dodges the issue, he is a poor doctor. Seek an alternative source. Check, also, any drugs the patient is taking. Blood pressure drugs, sedatives and antidepressants can all affect libido.

If the problems are purely physical, they can usually be solved. Careful use of pillows, or a new position, can counter one-sided weakness and lack of balance. If the patient lies on his or her weak side, that helps balance and leaves the good arm free. If the weak side has lost sensation, of course, it is distressing and a waste of time to caress it. If genital sensation has been lost, there are plenty of other nice places to caress. People who have been married you years can discover erotic zones they never knew about!

If the stroke patient is a man, the woman may have to be more active. For some couples this is fine; for others, the man finds his new passivity humiliating. Some rather old-fashioned couples have rarely ventured beyond the kind of activity which produces children, and will find it very difficult or 'wrong' to improvise. The best hope, here, is that the crisis of the stroke may have broken down some long-held inhibitions against touching and intimacy. If this can be built on before it fades away again, there is hope.

This brings us to the psychological side. Sexuality is a deep human need, and its fulfilment lies along a range which starts with just feeling attractive and ends with orgasm. Many stroke patients feel unattractive. From the start, make sure the patient is clean and well-groomed. Then progression along the range is possible. For men, feelings of self-esteem and being in control are often the most powerful aphrodisiacs. So working towards control and independence is working towards sexuality, too. Being able to excite one's partner also aids self-esteem, and is very erotic in itself.

If the carer is the patient's spouse, he or she may also have lowered sexual feelings. Carrying out intimate tasks isn't very erotic and he or she may indeed find the patient unattractive. This is hardly surprising, and nothing to be ashamed of. Pretending to be someone else (a nurse) when carrying them out is a game which helps. It helps even more when the patient takes over these tasks himself.

Sexual problems are relationship problems. A stroke is likely to change a marriage relationship completely, and often to devastate it. Honest work on these problems is essential, whether you want a sex life or not.

But the commonest sexual problem is the simplest – sheer exhaustion in patient and carer. Sex is just one more reason for planning lots of rest periods for both parties.

Workbook 6

This whole section is a workbook, with many checklists of (i) suggested activities and (ii) ways to make them easier. Start putting the two together.

Use **Care planning** (pages 33–6) to sort out what to do, analyse the small steps which lead to doing them, try them out and see if they worked.

Celebrate any success – however small.

Analyse failures – you now have more information on how to succeed.

Make absolutely sure that plenty of what you choose to do is enjoyable. This applies equally to patient and carer. They should do enjoyable things separately, as well as together.

What you are doing now is building up into a way of life. Is it the best way of life you could possibly have? If not, why not? What can you do about it?

For a change of perspective, use the **How's it going?** quiz which follows. It may set you thinking about new things worth aiming at. Or it may be just an interesting fantasy which tells you something.

How's it going?

This exercise is for patient and carer. Ideally, each of you should do it separately – and then compare notes. It may also be useful for other family members. Do it from time to time, to help you notice changes. Is there something new that you now want?

Your life has changed in many ways. You are working hard to cope with these changes, but sometimes you need to stand back and see things clearly. These exercises will help you pinpoint your progress, explore your feelings – and identify needs and problems you are neglecting. Be as detailed as possible in your replies. Be specific. Don't stop at your first answer to any question: go on until you have run out of ideas. You may find that the problems you identify have quite a simple, practical solution. You may find some good things you had forgotten were there.

1 What would be my ideal life? Go into total fantasy — no expense spared, no 'that would be nice, but ... '

What does this ideal life include that my real life does not include?

Is this something that can be changed?

If it can't be changed completely, is there some small thing that can be changed?

What does my real life include that my ideal life does not include?

Is this something that can be changed?

If it can't be changed completely, is there some small thing that can be changed?

2 What is the best possible thing that could happen in the future?

What is the worst possible thing that could happen in the future?

3 What is the best thing that has happened in my life so far?

What is the worst thing that has happened in my life so far?

4 Which of the people I know (or know of) do I most envy?

Why?

Which of the people that I know (or know of) do I most pity?

Why?

5 What are my best personal qualities? What am I good at

What are my worst personal qualities? What am I bad at

6 What is the most important achievement of my life so far?

What would I like to achieve during the rest of my life?

7 What is the worst thing I have done in my life so far?

What is the decision I most regret?

What would I do differently if I had the chance again?

8 What are the good things about my current situation?
   What can I do to build on them?
   What are the bad things about my current situation?
   Which of them are within my power to change? Which
   of them could be changed by somebody else?

9 What do I like about my carer/patient? Have I ever
   told him/her about it?
   What do I dislike about my carer/patient? Have I ever
   told him/her about it?

10 If a stranger met me today, how would he describe
   me?
   If a stranger met my carer/patient today, how would
   he describe him/her?

8

OTHER PEOPLE

From the very first day of the stroke, you will be dealing with other people – professionals, relatives, friends, children, perhaps employers. From the very first day, you are going to *need* other people – for practical help, for specialist advice and for emotional support. Keep an eye open for likely people, wherever you are. Keep your ears open for offers of help – don't ignore them.

How to get the best from people

Other people are the most important resource at your command. You may as well know, right away, that you can expect a few surprises – good and bad. You will find out who your friends are! Some people are terrified of illness and disability. They know strokes are not infectious, but they just can't cope. They are reminded of their own mortality and their own weakness. They see it reflected in the patient, and they can't face up to it. Short of a course of psychotherapy or a degree course in philosophy, not a lot can be done for such people. But you can still ask them to help you with things which don't involve contact with the patient.

Some people are terrified of strokes in particular. They retain an old-fashioned image of twisted, deformed bodies — something that just doesn't happen any more, with proper care. Or they assume the patient is as good as dead already. One carer was furious to find that even her own relatives avoided her mother. 'We'd rather remember her as she was,' they said. Do check out with other people what their image of stroke is. If they seem a bit reluctant, despite your pep talk, don't put moral pressure on them to visit in the very early days, when few patients look like a good advertisement for the joys of stroke. Save them for later.

Ignorance creates fear. With luck, your hospital or community services will have supplies of leaflets about stroke. Ask, if there are none, get hold of some cheap or free ones from an organization such as the Stroke Association. It saves you endless explanations, and it should arouse people's interest in your rehabilitation programme. Get them hooked and they should be willing to help out. They will realize that stroke is not just a question of living with a hopeless situation, but of an interesting project which aims to win back the patient's quality of life. Emphasize that you are working against the clock to take advantage of the body's power to regenerate, and the whole thing begins to look quite exciting ...

It is as well to be prepared for fear and rejection. If it takes you by surprise, it can be absolutely devastating. Better to be a little pessimistic, and then the surprises will be pleasant ones. Better to use a little understanding when you first approach people than to find out about their fears when it's too late and they've been put off.

There will be pleasant surprises, for sure. Towers of strength will rise up in unexpected places. The same carer who was so hurt by her relatives' attitude found a neighbour who was a constant support and became a firm friend. She also found that she could always rely on a cup of tea and sympathetic encouragement from the bank manager!

Important tip
Right from day one, seek out local volunteers and groups/clubs – especially those that have a special interest in stroke, or speech, or disability. Here, you will find people who actually *want* to help, without having to be persuaded. And – blissfully – they will know something about the problems, so you won't have to explain all the time.

Early days

It is very important, both for patient and carer, to maintain their place in the outside world. In the first few days you are in crisis. Your chief feeling is probably sheer shock. Both of you badly need somebody to talk to, cry with, yell at. Unless you are very unlucky, people will appreciate that and be prepared to fulfil this role for you. Normal social barriers will have been broken down and it will be possible, and acceptable, to talk about things you wouldn't normally talk about, show emotions you wouldn't normally show, touch people you wouldn't normally touch. Don't cut yourself off. People really don't mind being used in this way. It is, after all, rather flattering to be asked to play the big, strong comforter. The barriers will go up again, soon enough – in yourself, as well as in other people. Reach across while it's still possible. You may discover friends you never knew you had, who will go on being friends in the future.

Another thing which a crisis creates is offers of help. 'Is there anything I can do?' is a phrase on everyone's lips. Don't be afraid to take up those offers. Don't waste your energy on 'being strong'. You need it for other things. People *like* to feel they're being useful.

At first, you'll need two things. The first is practical help. You'll want people to hold the fort at home and/or at work. You'll need people to do shopping and run errands. You'll need help in gathering information. Probably one of the most important information-gathering jobs you might like to delegate is the financial side.

For nearly everyone, a stroke is a big financial blow. Grants and benefits are available but they are not easy to come by. All over the world, 'cutting down on public expenditure' is in fashion. In practice, that means that it is made as difficult as possible to claim financial help. Many people who are entitled to benefits never get them: they haven't been told what's available, and they haven't the time or persistence they need to jump through all the hoops which are put between them and the prize. First applications are often turned down; second applications succeed more often than not. It is difficult to avoid the suspicion that this is a method used, quite routinely, to put off everyone but the most determined.

Professionals like the doctor, the social worker and the local benefits office will give you a start. Some of them will be charming, supportive and go out of their way to help. Others would like to do all these things, but haven't the time. Some just don't care. You need the skills of a detective to follow up clues about which benefits are relevant to your own case. You need the patience of Job. And you need to be pretty assertive.

These are all very good reasons to call in someone else to help. He or she will have more time than you. And he will find it easier to argue on your behalf than you will to argue on your own behalf. Nobody relishes making pleas for help, but it's a different matter making pleas on somebody else's behalf.

The second thing you'll need most in the early days is visitors. It is very important to keep up all your contacts, without a break. The carer and the patient should not lose the habit of being social animals.

Some patients are very prone to cut themselves off and retire into a safe little world of their own. If the world insists on coming to visit them when they're still too weak to argue, and their own barriers are down, it will be all the easier to stop that withdrawal from ever happening. Do be sensitive, though. The patient will not want anyone and everyone to see him while he is so vulnerable. Choose carefully, and ask him whom he'd like to see, if that's at all possible.

Some patients become very possessive about their carers. They hate being attended by anyone else, and they hate to see their carer gallivanting off to do her own thing and delegating her responsibilities to others. Again, this situation should be headed off in advance. Start as you mean to go on. Every carer needs her own time and her own space. It makes her a happier person and it makes her a better carer. Don't get sucked into a tight little one-to-one relationship. It will become a bored, jaded and possibly bitter relationship. You both badly need to retain some sense of a personal identity, some kind of independence. You are working towards living a normal life again. Normal life includes being apart, as well as together, a sense of separateness as well as a sense of security and belonging.

And what do visitors need? You'll want to make their visits as pleasant as possible, so that they will continue. There's one simple golden rule about this: give the visitor something to *do*. Often, they find it hard to know what to say and feel helpless, embarrassed — and very bored! They won't be willing to repeat the experience. If the patient cannot speak or understand, of course, it's a great deal more difficult for visitors.

But doing something with the patient is a different matter. You will find some starter ideas in Section 1, Section 6 and, perhaps for later on, Section 7. Visitors should be delighted to find themselves doing something concrete. They may well enjoy finding solutions to some of the practical problems, when carer and patient have run out of energy and ideas.

There is no reason, either, why visitors should not be let in on some of the secrets of therapy. A vitally important but fairly straightforward task is good positioning, explained in Section 3. It's a job which has to be done constantly (whether the patient likes it or not!) and, for many people, it's a fascinating new concept which they will enjoy finding out about.

Intelligent help with lifting, once you are at home, will also be invaluable. Big, strong men are nice to have around, and teenage boys will be particularly flattered to be asked to help in this way. But small, weaker people can be just as useful if they know what they are doing. The techniques are explained in Section 3.

Other, more intimate tasks should be delegated with a great deal more care — if at all. Patients desperately need to keep up their dignity and self-esteem. So you will probably find that giving drinks is about the limit. Feeding won't be a very dignified procedure if the patient needs a lot of help.

The key is to make sure the visitor knows what is going on. If there are perception difficulties which cause odd behaviour, do remember to explain. If there are problems with communication, make absolutely sure that visitors understand the basic good manners and tips outlined in Section 6. Some people really can be very insensitive about this, and a single bad episode can do lasting damage to the patient's morale and confidence. Assume that your visitor needs to have the basics explained, so that such problems are prevented.

Also, make sure that the visitors know how vitally important it is to make the patient as independent as possible, as soon as possible (whether he wants to be or not!). You don't want all your efforts to be undermined.

People mean well. They feel sorry for the patient, they want to help and they hate to see the patient struggle with a task they could so easily do for him. You are, hopefully, trying to curb your own urges to be over-helpful, and to curb the patient's urge to have things done for him. So you don't want other people doing things you know the patient should do for himself. The last thing you need is a patient who complains: 'Lizzie does this for me. Why don't you?'

A final tip: remember that stroke patients get very tired. Time rest periods so that the patient is in the best shape to enjoy his visitors. When you are putting together a daily routine at home (see Section 7) it may be a good idea to schedule regular 'visiting hours' when people can be sure they will be welcomed.

Soon, you'll no longer be acting as nurse, therapist and all-round care assistant. The patient will have mastered some basic skills, will be able to attend to more of his physical needs, amuse himself at times and entertain visitors by himself. You'll be starting to put together the elements of a complete new way of life. If all has gone well, that way of life will be full of social contacts and activities – just as it should be.

Relationships

Most patients and carers have families. Sometimes they share the same family life: they are husband and wife, or have continued to share a home as parent and child, brother and sister, friend and friend.

Sometimes, however, the carer also has a family of her own. Married women with children are often drawn into the role of carer. Single people have satisfying lives of their own (although relatives are often happy to assume they have more time on their hands than married people!). They, too, are likely to be prime candidates for the role of carer. Such carers can be very painfully torn between the demands of their patient and the demands of their own life. If they attend to one, they feel guilty about the other. They may find themselves ricocheting between the two, never feeling they are doing enough for either. Often, the solution adopted is for the patient to move in with the carer's family.

Whatever the set-up, the stroke will change it deeply. In a traditional man-and-wife set-up, there will be a change of sex role. If the wife is the patient, the husband has to do the housework. If the husband is the patient, the wife has to take over his responsibilities, which may include anything from car maintenance to getting a job. Older people will probably find this particularly difficult and disconcerting. Everyone will find it hard work! Do make sure you get help from the rest of the family. And make a careful check on the jobs the patient used to do, for things he or she could still help with. Cooking? Gardening? Repairs? Care of pets? If he criticizes the way you do his old jobs, it's easier to bear if you can understand how much he hates having to hand them over.

The dominant person in the partnership (husband or wife)

may be the person who has the stroke. Suddenly, he or she becomes the weaker half. Do not underestimate the ructions this may cause. The quieter partner becomes the main organizer and decision-maker, which can cause a certain amount of panic and worry at the new responsibilities. The former decision-maker's self-esteem will take a knock – the last thing that's needed. The new 'leader' should make sure to keep him informed, ask his advice and see that he makes any decisions he is still able to make. Even when he no longer has any use of language, there are ways to bring him in.

Even worse, for many couples, is one partner's new role as nurse, teacher, therapist and (in the eyes of the patient) nag and bully. One of two very important things is likely to suffer damage: either the relationship, or the programme of therapy.

There are no easy solutions here. The patient must be made to understand how important it is to keep the therapy going, so he has to be nagged as little as possible. He must be shown that he is still loved and respected, so he is not too humiliated and is given the confidence and self-esteem to work towards independence. The partner in charge may find it helpful to pretend, in her own mind, that she really is a nurse or a therapist. It's easier, then, to drop the role when the task is over and return to something nearer the old relationship. If the patient still has his sense of humour, he could be drawn into the game as well. Then he, too, can be a patient sometimes – and a husband at other times.

Many of these problems will also apply if the carer is the son or daughter of the patient. Suddenly, he or she has become much more like a parent. The adjustment will be equally difficult, and the advice will be equally helpful. But don't expect an easy ride. All these role reversals will make all kinds of emotions well up, and may revive old difficulties from the past.

It helps to know that all these problems are commonplace, normal – and very understandable. Use the advice in Section 4 on **Feelings**. And talk to other people – professionals, friends and anyone who's willing to shut up and listen. Just saying how difficult things are, and being heard, can be amazingly effective in lifting the load – even if the situation itself remains unchanged.

Juggling two homes

Often, a carer does not have the patient in her own home. She may avoid domestic friction, but finds herself paying the price in time, travel – and guilt at leaving the patient.

Identify and deal with the practical problems. Much of the advice in **If the patient moves in with you**, on organizing routines and basic ground rules, holds good for this situation. So does the advice to have a regular review of how things are working out in practice.

The wider family

In a crisis, all kinds of other family members are pulled in. The chief actors are usually the patient's brothers and sisters, or the carer's brothers and sisters. Plus matching husbands and wives.

As with other people, the carer must take advantage of lowered barriers to get everything that's available in the way of comfort, and offers of help. By taking on the caring role, she is relieving everyone else. In too many families, this is taken for granted and the carer may feel guilty for expressing needs of her own – or upsetting the nice, neat plan by wanting to change it later on.

Feelings can well up. Jealousy is a common one. The carer is jealous of other people's freedom. The other people can feel jealous of the carer's role, and the praise and gratitude it can attract. If another relative makes a rare visit, and the patient talks of nothing else for days, the carer can feel *very* jealous. These feelings need to be accepted as inevitable (they are exactly that) and talked out, using the ideas in Section 4.

Use the **Can I go on caring?** exercise as a basic checklist to explore who can do what. Extra costs, for instance, are a burden which must be shared around. Specific 'contracts' need to be made, to ensure that all needs are covered – including the carer's. As usual, you need to be absolutely clear about what is needed.

Distant family, for instance, can promise to take the patient for just a fortnight a year, to give the carer a break, and can send letters, postcards or cassettes at regular (agreed) intervals. People closer at hand can review *all* the little jobs to be done, from shopping to minding the patient for a short while, from changing library books to doing research on what help is available, financial and otherwise. Vague promises get put off or forgotten. Specific commitments lodge in the mind – and family members can make a point of tactfully checking with each other that promises are being kept. Never let anything drift.

The patient's point of view must, of course, be kept in mind, and checked out, like everyone else's, from time to time. He, too, has the right to change his mind if the agreed arrangements are found wanting. But the final decision – to care or not to care? – must be made by the potential carer and nobody else.

A good tip: before any final decision is made – even a temporary one – talk to other families and carers who are in your kind of situation. Find out from them about problems they didn't expect to have at the outset.

Another good tip: no carer takes sole responsibility for caring. She may have the main responsibility, but that includes organizing other people to help – and looking after her own needs as well as the patient's.

To care or not to care?

In the first shock of the stroke, it is easy to feel a rush of compassion (or guilt?) which makes the role of carer seem natural and inevitable. Everyone involved needs to look a little more carefully than that, before decisions are taken.

About the only workable reason for caring is love – the chance to pay back past kindness from the patient. If your love is not genuine, underneath the day-to-day upsets, the patient can feel it. Strong-willed patients, who hate to be a burden, might well prefer to be cared for by professionals. Each situation is different. But nothing is worse than a commitment which is based on an unreal view of the problem – emotional as well as practical.

Make no final decisions at the outset. Try to avoid irrevocable acts, like selling the patient's home, in the first few months. Whatever arrangement is decided on, this must be for a trial period only and everyone must be made to understand that – including any professionals involved. The trial period must have a time limit, with a commitment from all concerned to review it.

But the most important thing is to make sure that the carer who gets the main responsibility is both willing and able to carry it. This has to be examined in ruthless detail at the outset, and re-examined to make sure the original decision was the best one. The **Can I go on caring?** exercise is designed for both these purposes.

Families come together in a crisis, but can drift apart again. Relatives may be very happy that the carer role has gone to somebody else, and will not want to have that decision questioned in the future in case the role of carer becomes vacant again.

Make decisions; don't drift into them, or allow other people to direct the drift. Review decisions when circumstances change. The change might just be in somebody's feelings – it is still a real change. Nothing is for ever.

If a carer is not willing, or has ceased to be willing, nobody benefits. Least of all, the patient.

Can I go on caring?

Get the latest professional advice about the patient's condition, his needs (in detail) and the progress he is likely to make. Changes in your lifestyle are inevitable. Use this checklist to help you define what those changes are likely to be – and whether you are prepared for them. And use it to pin down the help that other people are willing to commit themselves to give. Use the same check list to review the situation from time to time. Have the problems changed? Can you still cope? Do you need more, or different, help? Do you want a completely different arrangement to be made? Don't try to give something that you can't give. Know your limits.

1 How do you feel about the patient as a person? How was your past relationship? Do you think your feelings are a good basis for caring?

2 How does your spouse or partner (if any) feel? Is he/she trying to conceal negative feelings? How was his/her previous relationship with the patient? Is he/she willing to help? Is he/she willing for you to give time to the patient?

3 What about other members of your immediate family? Ask all the questions set out above.

4 Are you short-tempered, impatient or unwilling to compromise and make adjustments?

5 What about other family members?

6 Do you have plans and dreams which will have to be given up in order to care for the patient? How do you feel about this?

7 What about other family members?

8 What's your attitude in general to old people, sick people, disabled people? Be honest. Your attitude will colour your feelings towards this particular patient.

9 What about the rest of the family?

10 Are you physically strong enough to cope with the likely demands? Can you count on help when you need it?

11 Do you know where you can get emotional support when you need it?

12 What about other family members? They'll need support too, but should not get it all from the main carer.

13 Are there any skills you need to learn? These could be anything from lifting technique to dealing assertively with unhelpful professionals. Identify the gaps, so that everyone can contribute.

14 What is your understanding of the progress the patient is likely to make? Can you live with that?

15 What about other family members?

16 What if the patient does not make the progress you

expect? Is there any situation you feel you really could not stand?

17 Do you feel able to express your own needs, and your own feelings?

18 What about other family members?

19 What are the unspoken ground rules of the household where the patient will live? Is he likely to understand and fit in? Have you thought about what to do if he does not?

20 What about money? Have you got a broad idea of how much is needed now? What might be needed in the future? Can you cope financially?

Where can the patient live?

An honest effort at the **Can I go on caring?** checklist may reveal that nobody in the family can summon up a genuine desire to care for the patient. He may never have been very popular with any of you. None of you may have the time. All of you may realize you cannot willingly give up as much as is needed. Better to find out now than later. Better to work out another plan than to waste energy wishing you were all saints.

The patient himself may prefer to live outside the family circle. Many people dread being a burden. If they have to be nursed or rehabilitated, many people would prefer to turn the job over to an expert and let the family remain the family. The patient may enjoy the sense of security, and the company, of a special home.

The options range from sheltered accommodation, with minimal support, for people who can more or less take care of themselves, to a full-scale nursing home with trained staff who can do what hospital staff do. Prices vary enormously, so you need to know that some homes are free of charge, and that grants are available towards places at fee-charging homes. Grants won't cover the very expensive homes. The very expensive homes can be very good indeed, but they can also be awful.

Check before you make any commitment. A trial stay should be possible, and this is the only real way to be sure.

It can be tiresome work finding out what homes are available, and checking them out. It is better, however, than trying to unravel a mistaken choice. The patient should see the home before the choice is made, unless there are very good reasons why not. It is very important to talk freely (in private) to residents who are already in the home. If staff don't seem keen for you to do this, it's a very bad sign.

However sensible the decision, and no matter how much everyone agrees it is the best thing, 'putting someone in a home' can be a painful thing to do and may cause guilt, resentment and all sorts of other emotions which will have to be discharged. Use the advice in Section 3.

If the patient moves in with you

First, make it clear to everyone – the patient, the family and the professionals, too – that you are going to have a trial period. This period may, realistically, have to be a very long one. Older people, in particular, may take a long time to regain functions and learn ways to adapt. But nothing is for ever.

Use the **Can I go on caring?** exercise every few months, for all the family members to get in touch with problems which are bubbling up and were not anticipated. The situation changes. People's ability to cope, changes. Nobody should get locked into old arrangements which no longer fit present circumstances.

Be sure to give the patient a room to himself. It's even worth sacrificing the living room if necessary. Take care when you choose which room is to be the patient's. He needs regular rest, but he doesn't need a completely quiet life, shut away in an upstairs room, ignored for much of the time, and/or generally over-protected.

Relatives are people, with the same fears and hang-ups about stroke and disability as everyone else. Be aware when they show up, and use the advice given on page 199.

The family may resent the time the carer has to spend with the patient. The carer should do everything she can to draw them in to the patient's programme of care. Heaven knows, she needs the help. She should grab the chance to give her children this experience, which will make them feel grown-up and responsible even if it curtails their freedom. They will benefit as much as she does.

Small children adapt very easily to change, and will probably get on well with the patient if things are found for them to do together. But some children can't cope easily – especially if the patient can't communicate well. Sometimes, they can go through a phase of rejecting the patient completely. The speech therapist can be a big help. Or you may be able to get a play therapist or counsellor. Your best bet is to be honest and give lots of information. But don't bear the whole burden yourself. Get help.

Teenagers, quite often, are the family members with the most active social life and may be used to a pattern where the family organization revolves around them. They won't much like the change. They may reject the patient, in subtle or not-so-subtle ways. Consult them when decisions are made, ask them for help and explain, explain, explain. There is no reason why they should not know as much about the patient's condition and therapy as the carer. They will probably come up with some good ideas of their own. If they don't understand the principles behind the stroke patient's treatment, however, they will find his whole presence a bore.

Don't forget that teenagers can be squeamish creatures. They may find things like incontinence and eating problems very hard to take. Get expert advice on managing the incontinence if it lasts more than a few days. Muddling along could be disastrous. If the patient has eating problems, you're likely to find that he is keen to deal with them in private anyway, for the sake of his own dignity. Perhaps he could eat in his room and join the family for coffee.

A family routine will save shredded nerves all round. Even if you've been used to a happy-go-lucky lifestyle, it will be worth it. You'll be able to check that every single family member (including the carer) gets enough of the things he needs – togetherness and privacy, activities and rest, jobs to do and free time.

One thing you must balance carefully: as well as including the patient in the family's lifestyle, you must make sure he spends regular, predictable times in his room. The family must have time alone together, as they always have, and teenagers in particular might like to be assured the patient is in his own room if they have friends around. Do everything you can to make sure the family's social life doesn't suffer.

The patient can have visitors at any time, of course, in his own room. The smaller children will enjoy being his guests, and the patient could become a much-valued child minder. This will be good for him, and good for the rest of you. Encourage him to have his own visitors, too. A large piece of fabric draped over the bed, plus a few cushions, will turn it into an ordinary seating unit and make the room more like a sitting room than a bedroom. The patient's own

friends, if they are made welcome, are often more successful than the family in tempting him back to his old interests.

Don't underestimate the problems you all may face. The
patient will be upset at losing his own home. The upset,
and the loss of familiar surroundings, won't be much help
with his rehabilitation either. Cram in as many of his old
possessions as you can.

The family may or may not welcome its new member.
Nobody likes change, and arguments between generations
happen even when a stroke patient is not involved. Review
the situation from time to time as a family, and don't let
things drift. An outsider can be invaluable in helping you do
this. If you really try, and you conclude that the experiment
has been a failure, you have the right to hand back the
obligations you took on.

Getting someone in

Some carers need, or want, to go out a lot – to work, for
instance. Some may need to spend nights away from home.
And all carers need a complete break, as often as possible! The
simplest answer, often, is to have a paid carer to come in.

You may be able to manage with a patchwork of services
available locally or from the state: home help, visiting nurse
or care assistant, meals delivered, a neighbour popping in.
But it can be good to at least supplement all this with somebody *you* are paying, who is obliged to do what you want,
when you want it. For night-time care, you are almost certainly going to need someone to live in. If there's a particular
task that neither of you can learn to love, getting someone
else in to do it can be worth quite a heavy financial sacrifice.

Money, of course, is the problem. Check that the
allowances you get can be paid to a third party. Play on the

conscience of well-heeled relations who are not taking their share of the direct caring. Remember it is almost certainly worth paying out so that the carer can keep up his or her job. This will bring in income (if there's any left over after paying the paid carer), safeguard pension rights and safeguard the carer's independence.

Put out feelers through carers' group, patients' club, any professional you come across. There may well be a recently retired professional who would like a part-time job which uses her skills and experience. Advertise in the local venues – health centre, library, shops, any public building which allows it. Advertise in the local papers. Use an agency (but check their fees first, in detail).

Some rules of the game are:

- Put a telephone number in your ad if possible. It attracts more replies and enables you to do some preliminary sorting out with minimal trouble.
- Get somebody local if you can, so she does not herself become isolated.
- Sketch out the basics of the job right away to weed out the impossibles. Some people think caring for a disabled person is a light job, with lots of free time ...
- Line up some basic questions which fit the situation – can you lift someone constantly? are you a calm, relaxed type? are you willing to carry out therapy practice with the patient? do you like cats? Whatever.
- Make sure, in particular, that your paid carer understands the patient is an adult and will treat him as such, and that she appreciates the importance of making him independent.
- Leave patient and carer alone together at the interview, if possible.

- Take on any carer for an initial, clearly agreed, trial period. If the patient cannot speak, make special efforts to get feedback from him on how it is going.

- Give the new carer a clear list of what she has to do and when. If you are developing a set 'family routine' and diary (see Section 7), this is ideal. Demonstrate any techniques you use to lift or position the patient (etc) and leave this book as a reference. List, also, any strong likes and dislikes the patient has.

- If the patient has a communication problem, pay special attention to showing the paid carer how to cope with this.

- Sort out whether the paid carer will count as self-employed or as your employee. Try to avoid the latter, as it brings all kinds of complications like insurance stamps, tax administration and sick pay.

- Keep a note of everyone who applies. If one carer does not work out well in the end, others on the list may still be available months later. You may also need emergency cover.

- Remember that paid carers need a break, just like unpaid carers. Certainly there must be provision for holidays, and also for emergencies like illness. The ideal, for many people, is a rota of carers who know each other, can cover for each other when needed, can all work part-time – and can give the patient a constant change of faces!

- Remember that certain expenses like food, heating and telephone, may rise sharply.

Relief care

Whatever pattern of life you have worked out, it should contain some total relief for the carer. Families can take the patient for a holiday, or come in to 'sit' regularly. Some state provision is very good, with clubs, day centres and even regular hospital stays laid on for very dependent patients. Sometimes this is not ideal: low staffing means the patient does not get enough personal attention, and he may come back less independent than he went. On the other hand, time with the professionals can stop the rot if patient or carer have got stuck at a level of helplessness/over-protectiveness which is no longer justified. A word from an expert may convince, when nothing else would work.

There may, of course, be all sorts of emotional hangups connected with relief care. The carer feels guilty at wanting to get away from the patient, feels it is an admission of failure, feels anxious that other carers will show up deficiencies in her own care – or, conversely, may fail to keep up her own high standards. She may feel bitter towards the family for not offering more support; conversely, she may feel forced to accept offers of care from the family, even when they work out badly in practice. She may simply have forgotten what there is for her to do when the patient is not there. If the carer has reached that stage, she should redouble her efforts to provide some relief. She's on the edge of losing her whole identity.

The patient may be unwilling to be cared for by anyone else, and unwilling to leave home even for a day, let alone a longer stay. The danger is greater if you have not made efforts to keep up a social life from day one. He may exert pressure, subtle or not so subtle, which makes the carer give up the whole idea. Or, if he goes out once, he may make such a fuss on his return that the carer decides it is not worth it. This kind of thing is a major problem. It cannot, and must not, be put up with for long or the result is a resentful, bitter and burnt-out carer.

Intervention by a third party is the best way out, and a professional may carry extra weight in the argument. Somebody has to convince the patient that the carer has rights; somebody has to convince the carer of the same thing. Try to understand the fears and feelings behind the thoughts of both patient and carer – insecurity, fear of being abandoned or supplanted, guilt, resentment, lack of confidence, over-protectiveness. The patient, in addition, may not even realize just how much strain he is putting on the carer, unless somebody explains.

Relief care is not a mark of desperation. It is a normal human requirement. It should never be left until the last minute, when the situation has somehow become desperate. Find out what's available, from the start. Plan it into your normal daily life, from the start. Here are some tips:

- Check exactly what is on offer, and in particular what it costs. Some respite care is free, some is heavily subsidized, some is not.
- What other patients/residents will be the patient's companions? Will they be compatible, especially in age and in degree of handicap?
- Visit the facility in advance if you possibly can, preferably with the patient, and read the section on page 212 called **Where can the patient live?**
- Be bold. It's not unknown for a patient to be sent off, protesting bitterly, and return home having had a thoroughly good time. The transformation may not take place the first time, so don't give up straightaway.

- Start gradually. You may be able to go with the patient and stick around for a while. You may be able to keep in contact by phone (some places discourage this, and it's not necessarily a sinister sign – just an insistence that carers get a total break).
- Don't jetison other types of support if the relief care seems to work out. You need them all.
- Be aware that some relief care is so much in demand that you may not be able to have it for ever.
- Be aware that needs change. What is fine today may not be fine later on.

Workbook 7

This section contains a lot of information and checklists which should help you make decisions and plan actions. Make note of any idea that strikes you. As usual, choose the easiest thing to do first.

Some of these decisions and actions are bound to cause strong emotions. Look back to Section 4.

9

RESOURCES

This section is to be used at any time you need help. It may be useful on day one. It may be useful months later. Your needs will change, and it may be worth flicking through from time to time to see if any new ideas come to you.

It's also worth flicking through with the future in mind. As the patient progresses, more things become possible – what can you plan towards? Or a new crisis may come up – what new help do you need?

If you find out about all the help you can get, and use it right from the start, you are more likely to stop a crisis from happening. And you will be better able to enjoy all the good things which you could do.

RESOURCES ROULETTE

Strokes are very common, and take up a lot of health service time and money. But, often, not enough is done to plan for good stroke care, to earmark the proper resources for it, or to co-ordinate what *is* being done.

Because of this, it is almost impossible to give really detailed advice on what is available. It varies greatly from place to place, both in quality and quantity. There will be gaps. Or you may find that what is available is not tailored to your individual needs – wrong time, wrong place, too expensive, or in some way not quite what you had expected. For many people, transport is a major headache.

Of course, you are equally likely to find good care, supportive services and helpful people. Most people want to do their best to help – but they need to be told exactly what you need. Most professionals take pride in giving clients what they need – but not all of them have detailed knowledge of stroke.

Try to be clear about exactly what your problems are. And don't be shy about asking for help with them.

CATCH 22

This is the tricky thing. How can you ask for something if you don't know it exists? You are not an expert on stroke. There are all sorts of grants and benefits available, but state agencies will not go out of their way to tell you about them. There are all kinds of aids and equipment which could solve an irritating problem, but you can't be expected to know all about them.

There's no perfect answer to this. The first thing you can do is simply to define what your problem is. It could be: 'With both of us at home all day, the heating bills are worrying'. It could be: 'I can't wash my left armpit for myself'. Write down all the things that worry you, large and small, so you have a clear list.

Then – ask somebody who knows more than you do. In most cases, you can at least make an educated guess about the most suitable professional or agency. If you haven't a clue, ask *any* professional you are in contact with, or get in touch with one of the voluntary agencies. The person you first approach may not have the answer, but he or she may be able to suggest who does. If you know the problem, you can work your way towards the answer.

MONEY

Lack of money will make any kind of problem worse. Just as with services for stroke, financial help will vary from place to place, and from agency to agency. This is something you will need to sort out right from the start.

There is no reason to be embarrassed about finding out what you could get – and there is good reason to be determined about getting it. By caring for someone, you are saving the state millions. One British survey (by the Family Policy Studies Centre in 1986) calculated that the care provided by 1.3 million carers was worth up to £7.3 *billion*. You are fully entitled to support.

It may well be difficult to get. 'Cutting public expenditure' happens to be in fashion. Financial help is being cut all the time, in small ways and in big ways. You will have to *prove* your needs, and quite often to argue for them. If you apply for something and you are turned down – appeal. Appeals succeed more often than not. Refusing first applications seems to be almost a routine way to make sure that people don't get money unless they make a fuss.

Get into the habit of noting your expenses – large and small. Get into the habit of knowing *exactly* what your financial problems are. Get into the habit of asking about financial help, from any professional or agency you come in contact with. No one source will have all the answers. People won't always think to tell you all they know. Often, it will be up to you to take the initiative.

All this may be time-consuming, or even humiliating. It could be a good idea to turn over some of the detective work to somebody else, for example a sympathetic professional, a relative or friend. They will find it easier to argue on your behalf than you will to argue for yourself. Professionals are especially valuable, as their opinions carry weight with the powers that be.

Getting financial help is one of the responsibilities of caring. Don't allow anyone to see it any other way. Somewhere, you will find somebody who really is prepared to help – in the local Social Security office, the social work department, the hospital, a national organization. Find that help and use it!

WHO DOES WHAT?

This is perhaps the most confusing thing. The jobs of professional workers are fairly clearly mapped out, but they do overlap a bit. The same professionals might be employed by different agencies, depending on where you live – the hospital, the community health services, the social or welfare service or even a voluntary group or charity. It will be up to you to find out the strengths and weaknesses of the different agencies in your own locality.

You will also have reason to pick and choose between similar professionals. The patient, or the carer, may simply get on better with one particular professional – a purely personal thing, but it makes a difference. Or one particular professional may simply have a special interest in stroke – so his or her department becomes an extra-special resource, to be used to the full. Some splendid centres of excellence can arise in the most unexpected places.

Where you find a gap, the voluntary sector may fill it very well. This section lists several national charities who can open up a whole world of possibilities to you. Very often, they have local branches and clubs. Very often too, they can put you in touch with smaller organizations, which exist in their hundreds to fill specialist needs, or with small manufacturers who make a piece of equipment which is exactly what you want.

If you have any money to spare, you can fill some gaps with that – anything from taxi services to a private nurse or therapist. The telephone book will be a good source of information, and so will professionals and voluntary groups. Sometimes just an hour or two of paid help can make all the difference; sometimes you can buy better or more attractive versions of the equipment you are offered free of charge. Just make sure, before you spend anything, that you are not buying something you could get for nothing.

THE DOCTOR

When a stroke patient is in hospital, the hospital consultant is in charge of his care, although he may delegate some of the work to a junior doctor. Some hospitals have special units for stroke and/or rehabilitation. Others place stroke patients in various wards – geriatric, neurological, medical or even surgical. The consultant in charge is the one who controls the bed the patient is in. He is responsible for diagnosis, treatment (if any) and for making sure the patient has the nursing and therapy he needs. (Nurses and therapists are professionals in their own right, however, and a good consultant will delegate the appropriate responsibilities to them.)

When a stroke patient is cared for at home, the family doctor takes on the same responsibilities and is the gateway to obtaining help from nurses and other specialists – either home visits or appointments at the hospital outpatients department.

A good doctor can be very useful. She can tell you exactly what is wrong in your particular case (although a therapist will be more use in telling you exactly what the patient can and cannot do in terms of everyday activities). She can tell you about all the different kinds of help available, and her opinion will be crucial in helping you get everything you need. Not all doctors are specialists in stroke, so remember they may not have the last word on every problem. But they are, at the very least, an excellent starting point.

THE NURSE

Nurses, these days, do a lot more than just carry out doctors' orders. They are specialists in their own right. In hospital, they are the professionals who spend most time with the patient. They observe his medical condition and keep the doctor informed. They work closely with all the therapists, to make sure that early rehabilitation work is appropriate and consistent.

Some hospitals have specialist stroke nurses, although these are very rare in the UK. But all hospital nurses have specialist expertise, such as the prevention of pressure sores. And all nurses are supposed to take account of the patient's total needs – not just his medical conditions, but his feelings, hope and fears.

Outside hospital, there are nurses with extra training which helps them tailor their care to the individual situation – both emotional and practical. They have various names, such as district nurse, community nurse, health visitor, or visiting nurse. They may work for the health service, the social services or a voluntary organization. Most of them are 'hands-on' nurses, although some give advice rather than practical care. All these nurses should be a fund of practical tips, and of advice on what other help is available in your locality.

Some nurses have extra training and can give extra

services – advice on coping with incontinence, specialist help with physical handicap, counselling for emotional problems or psychiatric help. If you have a special problem, ask your visiting nurse if there is someone who can help.

The physiotherapist or physical therapist

Physiotherapists have specialized training about the body in movement – joints, muscles, bones, the effects of gravity and so on. Their aim is to make the patient as independent as possible, not to do things *for* him. Regaining the power of movement can be done only by pushing the body beyond its current limits, so they have to encourage patients to work hard.

Good advice from a physiotherapist is the key to maximum recovery of movement. At first, the patient must be placed in the right positions, or further damage will be done and maximum recovery will be made impossible. The physiotherapist should be called in straightaway to make sure this is done. Just as important, the physiotherapist knows about ways of lifting that are safe for the carer. Make sure you get advice on this.

Later on, the physiotherapist advises on the correct ways to get the patient moving. The wrong ways will be unsafe both for the patient and for the person who is helping him. As the patient progresses, individually tailored advice becomes more and more important. Learning to walk again is a tricky business.

Physiotherapists work for hospitals, community health services and social work agencies. If the patient is not in hospital, they may be able to make home visits. Otherwise, they will continue their rehabilitation work at outpatients' clinics or at daycare units.

It's a good idea, by the way, to show your physiotherapist this book. He or she will see the methods you are trying to follow, and may well be able to add some extra tips. The physio will also know much more about this individual patient than any book can, so may have some changes to suggest.

The speech therapist or speech pathologist

Speech and language therapists are, perhaps, the specialists who are least understood by other professionals. They have specialized knowledge of the brain, the effects of different types of brain damage, the workings of the muscles which control speech, and the way language is used and understood.

Traditionally, they have concentrated a lot of their efforts on children. Traditionally, also, it has been thought that they can do very little for adult stroke patients with dysphasia/aphasia. But research increasingly shows they can do quite a lot. For one thing, language recovery seems to go on well beyond the first period of spontaneous recovery – but only if speech therapy work is closely tailored to the patient's individual problem.

Speech therapists, however, do more than concentrate on words. Their job is to help the patient *communicate* – with or without actual words, using whatever means of expression he has. These alternative methods can achieve a very good level of communication.

Speech therapists work for health services, voluntary organizations and social work agencies. They may offer therapy one-to-one or in groups, weekly or in intensive blocks. Many, these days, run 'speech clubs' where several patients can socialize and practise together. They can teach family and volunteers to help each individual patient make the maximum progress possible.

Because their effects are sometimes undervalued, it can be difficult to get speech therapy. It is worth specifically requesting such help, to make sure it is given, and getting speech therapy privately if this is absolutely necessary. Action for Dysphasic Adults and the National Aphasia Association can help both to obtain speech therapists and to find ways to supplement their work.

The occupational therapist (OT)

These professionals tend to be in very short supply – so use them well! They need your help in getting to know the real needs of both patient and carer, so they know where to concentrate their efforts.

OTs may work in hospitals or in the community. The job is *not* to keep patients 'occupied' by making baskets or fluffy toys. It is to help people with disabilities to lead as normal a life as possible and to become independent.

The first priority is to help with basic things like washing, dressing, going to the lavatory, eating and getting around. Their input may include advice on adaptations to the home, teaching new methods to cope with specific tasks and recommending small 'aids' (like special cutlery) to make things easier. They can obtain many things for you, and give advice on others, including help with expenses.

If time allows, OTs can help with less 'essential' (but still very important) activities such as hobbies. There are specialists such as art therapists, craft therapists, music therapists, social therapists, drama therapists – if you can get one.

OTs tend to be 'hands-off' workers. They don't do things *for* patients and carers, but give technical know-how for people to do things themselves. They are trained to appreciate that psychological outlook is more important to progress than the degree of handicap, so they can give advice on motivation and morale. They look at the patient as a whole person – and give equal attention to his carers.

The social worker

Social workers come in all kinds of varieties. Some are 'generic' – trained to give help to just about anyone, on the reasoning that many families will have more than one member in need and they all have to get on together. Other social workers have specialist training – in mental health, for instance, in physical handicap or in working with carers.

A prime responsibility is to give advice on sources of finance. For many people, this is the most important help they can give. Social workers are also usually trained in counselling, so they should be able to take in the full meaning of what you say and should be able to identify the needs of the whole family – which, after all, affect the needs of the patient. In other words, they should be able to give emotional as well as practical support. And they should be a mine of information on all the facilities available locally.

Social workers work in hospitals, community health services and social work agencies. You may not be automatically referred to one, so if you think a social worker could help – ask.

Help with emotional problems

No single profession is the obvious choice here. Often, the most helpful person is simply the one you find it easiest to talk to, and who is willing to take time to really listen –

whether it's the nurse, the doctor or the woman next door.

Hospital chaplains can be very helpful, and you may not have to belong to their particular religion to see them. Local priests and clergy are also good to talk to – and may be able to organize all kinds of help, too.

Then there are all kinds of other specialists. You don't have to be mentally ill to see such people, and it is not a sign of weakness. Even the police, these days, recognize that nobody can be John Wayne all the time, and organize special support for employees under stress.

Such specialists can be obtained both through hospitals and through family doctors, as well as through social services. You may have to contact somebody privately, and in that case the American Holistic Medical Association or the Institute for Complementary Medicine should be your initial starting point in finding somebody properly qualified. In the USA, many such people have a social work qualification.

Psychiatrists train as doctors before going on to specialize in psychiatry, so they often (but by no means always) see their work as preventing or curing mental illness rather than as just talking people through their problems. Community psychiatric nurses may work for psychiatrists – or in their own right. Psychologists are not doctors, but their area of work shades into that of psychiatrists. Counsellors are trained to focus fully on what you say, and help you get in touch with your own hidden strengths to solve your own problems. Psychotherapists go rather deeper into your mind and your background, and some of them have extra skills such as hypnotherapy.

All these professionals work in the same kind of area – the mind and the emotions. They work according to many different schools of thought. The first person you consult may not turn out to be the right one for you, and you should not feel you are a failure if things don't work out.

Try someone else. Stroke is an emotional business, for all concerned. Even if you feel you are coping quite well, some extra help could make a lot of difference.

Volunteers and clubs

This area of activity has grown by leaps and bounds in the past few years. So there's a very good chance that you will find some kind of local volunteer service, or group or club. There is great variety, but you can be sure of being in contact with people who understand something about your situation – and are keen to help!

Both patient and carer will be able to meet people who are in the same boat. The patient, for once, won't be the only person in the room who can't speak or can't move easily. He may find people who are much worse of than himself – which can be good for the soul. The carer, for once, will be with people who know about stroke and/or the job of caring. She won't have to explain every little thing. She may be able to share a good moan – or even find a solution to a common problem.

There are all kinds of variations. There are groups for carers. Groups like the Red Cross can give (trained) emergency nursing care and respite care. There are day centres and clubs, run sometimes by state services and sometimes by voluntary groups. Often, the two work closely together.

In the UK, the Stroke Association funds some family support workers who visit people's homes, a day centre specially for young stroke survivors, an experimental 'advocacy' project to support people in claiming services and benefits, and a strong network of volunteers who visit patients with dysphasia, to help them practise their social and communication skills. They also run clubs for patients to get out of the house and meet each other. A similar scheme is run in the UK by ADA (Association for Dysphasic Adults).

The thinking behind all these schemes is developing as rapidly as the schemes themselves. For patients, the emphasis is no longer on doing things for them — but on giving them the confidence to do things for themselves. The goal nowadays is for the stroke survivors to run their own clubs. And for the clubs to encourage them to do as much for themselves as possible.

Find out what's available in your locality, by asking the professionals you meet and by contacting the national organizations listed in Section 9, **Resources.**

Note: volunteers and clubs provide a whole new dimension of life. What they can't do is replace the skilled work of professionals like speech therapists and physiotherapists. You need both. Volunteers and clubs may help patients to practise certain skills (under the supervision of a therapist). Or they may not aim to enter that area at all, but just to provide some stimulation and some fun. Either way, they are not a direct replacement for therapy. Don't be fobbed off by a state service that tries to kid you that they are.

Self help

In the end, you may find that the best way to get exactly what you need is to organize it yourself. This may not take an enormous amount of work, and may be easier (and less dispiriting) than wrestling with a service which can't or won't adapt to fit you.

Your best support will be a group of people who are in the same boat as you are. You are quite likely to find, locally, a stroke club, speech club, a carer's club or a local branch of a relevant voluntary group. Join it, whether you are a patient or a carer. At best, you will find that some-body has found the solution to your problem. At worst, you will at least have a fellow sufferer to grumble with.

If you can find no such group, organize one. This may seem like a daunting task but there are a lot of publications which can give you advice. Your best starting point is listed under **Support for carers** in section 9, and the national organizations listed under **Specially for stroke**.

One of the professionals you are in contact with may be willing to put you in touch with people in a similar situation to your own – whether you're a patient or a carer. And a professional's support will open many doors for you – even financial ones! A letter to the local paper could get a good response – or ring the features editor and suggest a whole article about the need for a club or group. Local radio will also get you useful publicity. Local media are usu-ally very helpful to local people who can give them a 'human interest' story.

You need only one reply from a like-minded person to give you the energy to take things further. After a certain point, the project will acquire an energy all of its own, and little bits of help will start to turn up.

There are all kinds of local groups which will be able to provide help, in cash or in kind; places of worship and their congregations, Scouts and Guides, schools, youth groups, Rotarians, Elks and the like, community centres, ex-servicemen's groups, ex-employers, local firms looking for some good public relations outlets. Start with someone you know.

As always, the first task is to define exactly what you need. Then break it down into small steps – and see who is willing to give some small thing, or a little bit of time.

People really do like to help. What holds them back is

not knowing what help is needed, or fearing that they will be asked for too much. Define what you need, take it gently and keep your eyes open. Once you start looking, you may be surprised at the possibilities you see.

But the first step has to come from you.

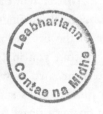

USEFUL ADDRESSES

Loads of help is available, if only you can find out where to look. This list can only be an indication of the hundreds of contacts that can help you with anything from Black disability issues to wheelchair water-skiing.

The list is divided into sections: specially for stroke, money, therapy, support for disabled people, support for carers.

If you've got a problem, decide which of these sections seems the most relevant. Then have a go – try someone on the list. If they can't help, at least they are likely to know who can!

If you really haven't a clue where to start, try the organisations 'specially for stroke'. If your problem looks hopeless and there seems to be no point ringing anyone, again ring a stroke organisation.

Specially for stroke

All these organisations are your gateway to: lots of useful publications, telephone advice, local branches, volunteer helpers and clubs for both stroke survivors and carers.

UK

Stroke Association, CHSA House, 123–127 Whitecross Street, London EC1Y 8JJ. 0171 490 7999.

Action for Dysphasic Adults, 1 Royal Street, London SE1 7LL. 0171 261 9572.

USA

National Stroke Association, 8480 East Orchard Road, Suite 1000, Englewood, CO 80111–5015; (800) 787–6537; (303) 771–1700.

American Heart Association, 7272 Greenville Ave, Dallas, TX 75231–4596. (800) 242–8721; (800) 553 6321 STROKE CONNECTION; (214) 373–6300.

AUSTRALIA

Australian Brain Foundation, 746 Burke Road, Camlewill, 3124 Victoria. 03882 2203.

Money
UK

Your local Citizens Advice Bureau

Your local Social Security office

Your regional Disability Benefits Centre (look in the phone book or ring the Benefits Agency, 0171 962 8000).

Freeline Social Security: 0800 666555 or (Northern Ireland only) 0800 616757.

Benefits Enquiry Line (specially for disability benefits): 0800 882200 or (N.Ireland only) 0800 220674.

Disability Alliance, 1st floor east, 88–94 Wentworth Street, London E1 7SA. 0171 247 8776. Rights Advice Line 0171 247 8763.

Disablement Income Group, Unit 5, Archway Business Centre, 19–23 Wedmore Street, London N19 4RZ. 0171 263 3981.

National Debtline 0121 359 8501.

USA

Medicare information: American Society of Internal Medicine, 2011 Pennsylvania Avenue, NW, Suite 800, Washington DC 20006. (808) 835–2746.

National Health Information Center, US Department of Health & Human Services, PO Box 1133, Washington, DC 20013–1133; (301) 565–4167; (800) 336–4797.

Healthcare Financing Administration, US Department of Health & Human Services, 6325 Security Boulevard, Baltimore, MD 21207;

MEDICARE HOTLINE (recorded) (800) 638–6833.

Social Security Administration, Office of Public Inquiries, 6401 Security Boulevard, Baltimore, MD 21235. (800) 772–1213; (410) 965–7700.

AUSTRALIA
Your local Social Security office

Therapy
For general advice on what a certain therapy can do, and how to find a properly qualified practitioner.

UK
British Association for Counselling, 1 Regent Place, Rugby, Warwks CV21 2PJ. 01788 578328.

Chartered Society of Physiotherapy, 14 Bedford Row, London WC1R 4ED. 0171 242 1941.

College of Occupational Therapists, 6–8 Marshalsea Road, London SE1 1HL. 0171 357 6480.

College of Speech and Language Therapists, 7 Bath Place, Rivington Street, London EC2A 3DR. 0171 613 3855.

British Council for Complementary Medicine, PO Box 194, London SE16 1QZ. 0171 237 5165.

USA
Alternative/complementary therapies: Committee for Freedom of Choice in Medicine, 1180 Walnut Avenue, Chula Vista, CA 91911. (800) 227–4473. (619) 429–8200.

National Health Information Service, US Department of Health & Human Services, PO Box 1133, Washington, DC 20013–1133; (301) 565–4167; (800) 336–4797.

National Wellness Institute, 1045 Clark Street, Suite 210, Stevens Point, WI 54481. (800) 243–8694; (715) 342–2969.

People's Medical Society, 462 Walnut Street, Allentown, PA 18102. (800) 624–8773; 2150 770–1670.

American Occupational Therapy Association, 4720 Montgomery Lane, PO bOx 31220, Bethesda, MD 20824–1220. (301) 652–2682.

American Physical Therapy Association, 1111 N.Fairfax Street, Alexandria, Virginia 22314. (703) 684–2782 ext. 3143.

American Speech, Language & Hearing Association, Rockville Pike 10801, Rockville, MD 20852–3279. (301) 897–5700.

National Association for Hearing and Speech Action, 10801 Rockville Place, Rockville, MD 20852. (301) 897–8682; CONSUMER HELPLINE (800) 424–2460.

AUSTRALIA
Australian Association of Occupational Therapists, 6 Spring Street, Fitzroy, Victoria 3065. 03416 1021.

Australian Association of Speech & Hearing, 212 Clarendon Street, East Melbourne, Victoria 3002. 03419 0422.

Australian Physical Therapy Association, PO Box 6465, Melbourne, Victoria 6465. 39534 9400.

Support for disabled people
These organisations, most of them charities, can provide all kinds of telephone advice, publications and local contacts, covering everything from financial help to holidays. If the one you happen to ask can't help, it will know who can. It will probably also be able to give you a local contact.

UK
Association to Aid the Sexual and Personal Relationships of People with a Disability, 286 Camden Road, London N7 OBJ. 0171 607 8851.

Continence Foundation, 2 Doughty Street, London WC1H 2PH (Helpline 0191 213 0050).

Disabled Living Centres Council, Winchester House, 11 Cranmer Road, London SW9 6EJ. 0171 820 0567.

Disabled Living Foundation, 380–384 Harrow Road, London W9 2HU. 0171 289 6111.

Help the Aged, St James's Walk, London EC1R OBE. 0171 253 0253. Freephone advice 0800 665544.

RADAR (Royal Society for Disability and Rehabilitation), 12 City Forum, 250 City road, London EC1V 8AF. 0171 250 3222.

USA

American Rehabilitation Association, PO Box 17675, Washington DC 20006. (202) 737–8300.

Help for Incontinent People, PO Box 544, Union, SC 29379. (800) 252 3337. (803) 579–7900; also: Simon Foundation, PO Box 815, Wilmette, IL 60091. (800) 237–4666; (708) 864–3913.

Information Center for Individuals with Disabilities, 20 Park Plaza, Room 330, Boston MA 02116. (800) 462–5015.

National Association of Area Agencies on Aging, 1112 16th Street, NW, Suite 100, Washington DC 20036. (202) 296–8130; to find out your local agency, call ELDERCARE LOCATOR – (800) 677–1116.

National Organization on Disability, 910 16th Street, NW, Suite 600, Washington, DC 20006. (202) 293–5960; (800) 248–2253.

National Rehabilitation Information Center, 8455 Colesville Road, Suite 935, Silver Spring, MD 20910–3319. (301) 588–9284; (800) 346–2742.

National Council on the Aging, 409 3rd Street, SW, 2nd Floor, Washington, DC 20024. (202) 479–1200; (800) 424–9046.

AUSTRALIA

Disability Information & Resource Centre, 195 Gilles Street, Adelaide, SA 5000. (08) 223 7522.

Disabled Peoples International (Australia), 30 Storey Street, Curtin, ACT. (06) 282 3025.

House With No Steps (Wheelchair & Disabled Association of Australia), 49 Blackbutts Road, Belrose NSW 2085. (02) 451 1511.

Independent Living Centre, 46 Canning Street, Launceston, Tas 7250. (003) 34 5899.

Macarthur & District Association for the Disabled, 9 Broughton Street, Campbelltown, NSW 2560. (046) 26 8500.

Rocky Bay Inc (for children & young adults only), 60 McCabe Street, Mosman Park, WA 6012. (09) 384 1855.

Tasmanian Association of Disabled Persons Inc, 112
Gormanston Road, Moonah, Tas 7008. (002) 72 0222.

Technical Aid to the Disabled, 227 Morrison Road, Ryde, NSW
2112. (02) 808 2022.

Victorian Advisory Council on Recreation for People with
Disabilities, PO Box 55, Carnegie, Vic. (03) 9666 4200.

Yooralla Society, 52 Thistlethwaite Street, South
Melbourne, Vic 3205. (03) 9254 5666.

Support for carers
UK
Back Pain Association, 16 Elmtree Road, Teddington,
Middlesex TW11 8ST. 0181 977 5474.

Carers National Association, 20–25 Glasshouse Yard,
London EC1A 4JS. 0171 490 8818.

Crossroads Care Attendant Scheme, 10 Regent Place, Rugby
CV21 2PN. 01788 573653.

Family Service Units, 207 Old Marylebone Road, London NW1
5QP. 0171 402 5175.

National Council of Voluntary Organisations, Regent's Wharf,
8 All Saints' Street, London N1 9RL. 0171 713 6161.

USA
There is no known organization at national level specifically
for carers, so see what you can find via the organizations for
disability and stroke.

US Red Cross, 17th & D Street, NW, Washington DC 20006.
(202) 728–6600.

AUSTRALIA
Australian Red Cross, 206 Clarendon Street, E.Melbourne,
Victoria 3002. (3) 941 85200.

Carers Association of Australia, PO Box 3717, Weston, ACT
2611. 06 288 4877.

Carpenteria Respite Services, 45 Henbury Ave, Tiwi, NT810.
08945 4977.

INDEX